STIR IT UP

Commercial Nonfiction

A Tourette syndrome Case Study
& Social Commentary by

Parrish Douglas

Published by
D.P. Media International
Copyright © Parrish Douglas, 2001 - Clinically Frustrated   TXu 1-025-482
Copyright © Parrish Douglas, 2010 – Stir It Up

LIBRARY OF CONGRESS CATALOGING-IN-PUBLICATION DATA:
ISBN 978-0-615-31293-4

Printed in the United States of America
Set in Dexter, Michigan by Thomson-Shore
First Printing, July 2010
Designed by Parrish Douglas

2 TIMOTHY 2: 23-25

English Standard Version

"Have nothing to do with foolish, ignorant controversies; you know that they breed quarrels. And the Lord's servant must not be quarrelsome but kind to everyone, able to teach, patiently enduring evil, correcting his opponents with gentleness."

Read the above passage over and over again as you stumble with my writings in this book. Understand that this work is my personal attempt at finality with these things that I do. Many of the controversies I see and hear in the media are foolish indeed; but most of mine are legitimate. When this is done I intend to go into the world and to leave it a better place.

~Parrish Douglas

Dillon,
Good Reading
+ good luck.

Most books are ghost written, which means to have a staff of people work on it and then to put it under the name of a more famous person for sales reasons. That person may have in fact had some ideas or some input. This is particularly the case with comedians and preachers. They write material for speech but they do not put it together on paper. They just use bullet-point notes. Somebody comes along later and edits the whole thing.

I want you to know that I refused all day long to tolerate this kind of process and that every last word in this entire book was penned and then edited by myself in an experience that lasted over 10 years. I love this book with all my heart. It is my masterpiece in oil paint, my symphony in F# augmented.

The placement and choice of every word is intentional.

You will see this Papyrus font and this color used when the author is quoting himself. I have also chosen to use different fonts to grasp your attention. I myself am a notoriously slow reader.

All the pictures were my idea. I took all the pictures myself except for the ones that I am in. Yes, some of the body parts might be mine too.

The only being that gets credit for inspiring my work is the Holy Spirit. Thank you and Amen.

TABLE OF CONTENTS
THERE IS JUST SO MUCH TO SAY ABOUT EVERY LITTLE SUBJECT IN EVERY CHAPTER THAT IT BECOMES DIFFICULT TO ORGANIZE IN A MEANINGFUL MANNER.

FOREWORD   15

PHOTO: STRAIGHT JACKET IN PARADISE
I   CLINICALLY FRUSTRATED   23
    A. THE WAY I SEE IT
    B. TS – TECHNICAL DEFINITION
    C. TRIGGERS
    D. TICS
    E. PSYCHOLOGISTS
    F. DREAMS

PHOTO: BODY SHOTS
II   GENERAL GRIPES AND BITCHES   39
    A. 13 RANDOM THOUGHTS
    B. REGULAR TELEVISION
    C. CHILDREN'S TV PROGRAMMING
    D. THE MOVIES
    E. SPORTS
    F. TURNING OLD
    G. HOMEWORK BEFORE SHOPPING
    H. THINGS CHANGE: ACCEPT IT
    I. MOVING INTO THE FUTURE
    J. TOO MANY CHOICES
    K. DON'T BE CHEAP
    L. DESIGNING YOUR LIFE
    M. HAIR REMOVAL
    N. HOMELESSNESS

PHOTO: ILLEGAL ALIENS

III   ALIENS AND U.F.O.'s   69
       A. GET READY 'CAUSE HERE THEY COME
       B. CLOSE ENCOUNTER
       C. GRAYS
       D. ACTUAL MARTIANS
       E. OTHER RACES
       F. NEW MEXICO
       G. ALIEN TECHNOLOGY
       H. COMMUNICATIONS DEVICES
       I. FOOD
       J. ALIEN RELIGIOUS BELIEFS

PHOTO: LEADERS OF TOMORROW

IV   GOVERNMENT AND LAW   87
       A. TALK SHOW BITCHES
       B. THE PRESIDENCY
       C. FORMING A ONE-NATION PLANET
       D. IT IS DONE
       E. CRIME IN GENERAL
       F. RETRIBUTION
       G. RAPE
       H. CAPITAL PUNISHMENT
       I. THE RACKS
       J. GRAFFITI AND LITTER
       K. FIGHTING
       L. TERRORISM

PHOTO: TOMATO GIRL SOUP

V   ECONOMY   111
       A. WAGES
       B. TAXES
       C. .95 .98 AND .99
       D. WASTE

E. REAL ESTATE
F. GREAT FOOD AND FREE FOOD
G. MEDICAL CARE
H. EDUCATION
I. INSURANCE

PHOTO: SPARE TIRE
VI   TRANSPORTATION   129
        A. ROAD CONSTRUCTION
        B. PUBLIC TRANSPORTATION
        C. AIRLINES
        D. ALTERNATIVE POWER
        E. MOVEABLE WALKWAYS
        F. BIG BUSINESSES
        G. BUILDING THE BETTER BEAST
        H. GOING TO THE CAR DEALERSHIP
        I. SPEED & THE DIAMOND LANE
        J. PAYING ATTENTION
        K. ART IN MERGING
        L. LICENSE REVOCATION
        M. DRIVING SCHOOLS
        N. AUTO INSURANCE SCAMS

PHOTO: NIPPLE SUITS
VII   EMPLOYMENT   149
        A. OPPORTUNITY
        B. EEOC
        C. HUMAN RESOURCES
        D. TO MARKET (VERB)
        E. METRICS
        F. GIVING RAISES
        G. CLEANING HOUSE
        H. THE REVOLVING DOOR EFFECT
        I. SEXUAL HARASSMENT

PHOTO: CREAMY SMURF
VIII RELATIONSHIPS   163
    A. THE PERFECT DATE
    B. CHEATING
    C. DIMINISHING A CAPACITY FOR LOVE
    D. DATING IN GENERAL
    E. STRANGERS
    F. HONESTY
    G. LOVE OR LUST
    H. LETTING THE SPARK DIE
    I. DECISION MAKING
    J. LEARNING TO LOVE
    K. THINGS TO DO TO KEEP IT FRESH
    L. FIGHTING WITH YOUR MATE
    M. BREAKING IT OFF
    N. REVENGE

PHOTO: FRENCH SILK PIE
IX SEX   197
    A. SEX FOR HETERO'S
    B. THE TOP 5 QUESTIONS
    C. UTERUSES
    D. MANANAS
    E. BREASTS
    F. HAVING AN ORGASM
    G. THE MAGIC WOO-WOO
    H. POSITIONS
    I. THE MISSIONARY STORY
    J. MY EXPERIENCE HAS BEEN...
    K. AFTER PLAY
    L. HORMONES
    M. THAT'S WHAT LITTLE GIRLS ARE MADE OF
    N. MASTURBATION
    O. GAYNESS

PHOTO: "CUBANOS BLANCOS"
X   REPRODUCTION AND CHILD REARING   223
          A. GOD'S ROLE
          B. THE GOVERNMENT'S ROLE
          C. PERMITS
          D. ABORTION AND ADOPTION
          E. CLONING
          F. RESPONSIBILITY
          G. CHILDREN IN PUBLIC
          H. METHODOLOGY IN PROBLEMS
          I. RESPECT AND TOUGH LOVE
          J. DISCIPLINE
          K. TEENAGERS
          L. SCHOOL

PHOTO: AIR PLAY
XI   THE CHOSEN PATH   249
          A. CHILDHOOD
          B. INDECENCIES OF YOUTH
          C. COLLEGE
          D. BECOMING AN ENTREPRENEUR
          E. BROKERS
          F. CURRENTLY

PHOTO: FATMAN FANTASY
XII   THEORIES AND THE SECRET OF LIFE   265
          A. CARPE DIEM / SEIZE THE DAY
          B. HONESTY
          C. SAYINGS TO LIVE BY
          D. THINGS TO SEE BEFORE YOU DIE
          E. PSALMS OF EL GRAN AMANTE
          F. PROVERBS
          G. VIRTUES AND SINS
          H. THEORIES

    I. ALL THINGS DRINKING
    J. TRAINS
    K. NUDIE BARS
    L. 2012 END OF DAYS?
    M. ....AND WHEN I'M DEAD, DEAD AND GONE

PHOTO: DO YOU SEE THE LIGHT?
XIII SPIRITUALLY MEDICATED   301
    A. FORMAL RELIGION
    B. BEING ONE WITH THE PEW
    C. TITHING
    D. PROFANITY AND HYPOCRISY
    E. CREATION
    F. PERSONAL STRUGGLES
    G. AFTERLIFE
    H. RE-INCARNATION
    I. WORLD RELIGION COMPARISONS
    J. MYTHOLOGY

PHOTO: MY SHADOW
XIV IN CLOSING – THE FINAL CHAPTER   337
    A. AS MY BOOK ENDS
    B. CREDITS AND COMMUNICATIONS
    C. LAST CALL

PREFACE

HOW WE MET...

I remember your smile and your hesitation that first day. I gazed upon your beauty from across the aisle. You were unaware that I had entered. You have always been beautiful and I thought, one day I must have this woman in my life. You were shy and fragile. I knew in an instant that you were different; a kindred soul. We began our journey.

WORDS IN RED

Some scholars do not like the red letter editions of the Bible.
They say this because both the exact words of Jesus have been
lost in translations over the years and because some believe that
all the words of the Bible are from God; penned by different
authors such as Paul. I agree with this but I like red for effect.

Anything quoted in my book from any bible -or- words that I think
God might say someday are in red.

I put my quotes in red because Jesus loves me.

Plus, the printing company charges a metric f**k-ton of money
to print in 4-color for the entire book so we might as well use it.

FOREWORD

Initially the title of this book was to be "Clinically Frustrated", which I thought was a brilliant title and one which more than accurately describes its contents. The better of me thought that people might be hesitant to take a book to the checkout line that said **FRUSTRATED** in big bold letters. Now that title belongs to a single chapter which in hind sight was added because it offers so much more clarity to the literary debacle that takes place before you now! Only part of this book is dedicated to my condition that I refer to as TS. The rest of the book is about my perceptions of things because I have TS and am frustrated. I want you to understand a different perspective. At any rate, one day I was discussing the book with my Aunt, and when I told her that the whole point of the book was to stir up controversy in peoples' minds and get them thinking about subjects in a different light. She suggested the current title "STIR IT UP".

This book is prophetic. The ideas I present will come to pass; many of them in your lifetime. You the reader might be the cause of great change. I hope to be your catalyst. The point of this book is to plant a seed in your mind. It is not that all of the things you read about are possible right now, but if I can open everybody's mind just a little more, anything can become a reality. It is my sincere hope that your mind will be forever tainted and that everything you see around you will have new meaning once you are finished reading and viewing my awesome photography. There are a lot of valuable insights within these pages, but some of them may seem a bit unorthodox at first. Would you call the late fiction writer Jules Verne a visionary? Many do, and for good reason. His writings sounded far-fetched. It's not fiction anymore is it? Vision is the hallmark of genius.

STAY ON THE ROAD

You should take notice that this book intentionally labels the first page as page 1 and that the sections one would normally pass over are not designated as a Roman numeral preface. I have always considered this practice in publishing to be absurd. They can print books and have lots of money, yet they cannot count correctly. That to me says that all the material that comes before chapter 1 should be labeled B.C., and everything after as A.D. The stuff in the beginning has equal validity. The content is just prefatory and prepares you for what is to come. They did insist that I have one page of blankness at the beginning and the end as a formality. Apparently it costs less to print hard back books with page numbers divisible by 8, so I had to push it to 344.

It is important that you read this introduction and not try to skip forward to the meat of the book. Some chapters will indeed be more outright entertaining than others, but please ignore the impulse for immediate gratification, savoring in the knowledge that the more juicy segments will abound when you least expect them! Much like your favorite CD, the tracks were put in a specific order for a reason. This is my work of art. Without an understanding of the author, one might formulate incorrect opinions based on a lack of knowledge. This is human nature. That statement is not intended to offend anyone, rather it is a statement of fact to say that as a race, we feel we can instantly assess a situation or information and correctly make a right judgment upon it. In fact, the majority of persons today are indeed close-minded, so I invoke you to open your minds and become a better being.

Our society is already rated R so keep that in mind when you read this. I am also writing this with the full knowledge that I will contradict myself many, many times.

What I would like for people to know is that I am quite healthy and sane. I would prefer not to be recognized or branded as a sick individual, rather as one who provided knowledge, insight and entertainment. Horror writers are not sick people, they are just doing a job, and so am I. This is my defense. Carry a copy of this book with you at all times. Share it with your friends so that they may learn as well. Don't laugh too hard at the sex chapter.

It doesn't really matter what anyone who reads this book thinks of me. It is not important nor is it a relevant issue in my life. I am thoroughly not impressed with the way most of you live and I believe that society needs both a large scale intervention and a liquid Enema. I would like to know that my message has had a future impact in the lives of many. This book is a life reference guide written and intended for people who feel they deserve to be in the upper crust of humanity if indeed there is such a thing; not at all divided by money or class but rather by intelligence and social competency. I would like for it to be considered as a classic work that is referenced in classrooms and conversations for generations to come. The book will probably mock you and your siblings at one point or another. Those with a fleeting mentality and the pension to act like "white trash" deserve nothing less. In addition, if you cannot take a joke, a punch in the stomach, or a tall strong shot (at least 1 of the 3), this book is not for you.

In the event that this book should become successful, I have purchased weapons and a large motor home and intend to disappear for a while on sabbatical. Humanity is overrated.

FRUSTRATION

The former title is a state of being, wherein one becomes angry at the world around them because nothing is as it is should be. You may feel this way because you were to have reached certain goals in your life that you have not achieved yet. These goals were obvious in your youth and the rewards were to be obligatory in the adult stages of our lives given that we performed certain tasks like making our way through college. The frustration comes about because we believe that someone or something has failed us. Not that we have failed ourselves because that is rarely possible in our minds eye. Our parents led us to believe in a standard and the fact that some of our friends have achieved that standard sends our minds into a downward spiral. It keeps us searching for answers when there are none. Is it because we were not taught early in life to wish for very little, and we were not given the tools and attentive guidance to achieve very much? Most of us do have the mental awareness, acuity and predisposition for greatness; we just need to be given a fair chance.

One contemplates their chances or lack thereof usually while resting. Bed (or a hammock) is one of the most wonderful places on Earth. It is like a sarcophagus, a recharging station for not only the body but the mind as well. I like that word, sarcophagus. I would like to decorate my daily resting chamber like one. A person should not be bothered while in their bed, even if you know someone who likes to lay in bed all day or one who hides in their bed to escape from their lives. Many of the world's foremost thinkers have historically taken naps at different times of the day or slept in late. It is because they need time away from the annoyances of every day life to contemplate how the world might be if they could change it. Frustration can also come from having to get out of bed too early. Your mind is brilliant when it is in this state of peace.

I have chosen to include a chapter toward the end about my life and experiences so that you can better relate yourself to me. Perhaps you can identify with similar situations in your life. As for the nature of the pictures that I took; well you would have done the same if you had the opportunity. Frankly I am surprised that all authors don't go off the deep end and include better visual stimulants.

"Photography is the art of telling a story by capturing one single moment in time." – You see, I wrote and immortalized that statement just now with the copyright of this work. You can use it for free if you want to, as long as you give me the verbal credits.

Why Am I Doing This?

Why publish what so many people will consider to be the most offensive literary work of all time if I know it is going to cause bitter arguments? The secondary answer is to help the rest of you. I do see the light. I understand the ebb and flow of life. I know exactly why I suffer on multiple levels. I also recognize that not one man is righteous. I need for you to understand that I felt it in my heart that I had to publish this work, but also that by doing so I am accomplishing the primary goal of publicly repenting for my sins. I am a sinful, shameful man. I repent on a minute-by-minute basis just like all of the Doobie Brothers. I want to be a better man but in order for that to happen I have to acknowledge that I am not good. My heart tells me what is right and it now tells me that after this is published I may pick up the pieces and try to help others see the light. That is my calling. I am also called to be a loving husband to a beautiful woman that deserves to be treated with kindness and to possibly help raise an adopted baby girl. Time will tell if that happens. I can hide nothing from my future wife. She has to accept me as I am and through transcendent love I will accept her also. I have other plans for life, sure. That's the plan that I believe God has for me. The rest is insignificant.

Finally I would like to thank you for selecting and reading this book. It is amazing to me the amount of determination, effort, research, and just plain work that goes into writing (and primarily editing) a book. It is an immense project to undertake. It's a little long but only because I wanted to get all of my bitching out in one novel. I do not wish to do this again. Your posture falls apart, and that probably adds to the end cost. The publisher has to pay the author more to supplement the lack of medical insurance and chiropractic care.

People told me that I couldn't write a book that covers so many different topics. A lot of publishers told me it was unmarketable. They were wrong. They just like to be very controlling over what they think you should read. I finished it anyway. Mostly out of spite.

I don't have lots of cash so I couldn't just take off work. It seems that the only time one can have a creative thought is in the middle of the night. So just try to write the great American novel if you're a working mom or dad or anybody working at all. The working class people are my heroes just because I lack the ability to do it the normal way. I wish you good luck in your lives. I hope you will find something here that stirs you to take up a pen and write about your passions. Maybe something you've always wanted to say, and to have the world hear. Thank you again for making a major part of this dream of mine become true. The honor is mine.

Parrish ~

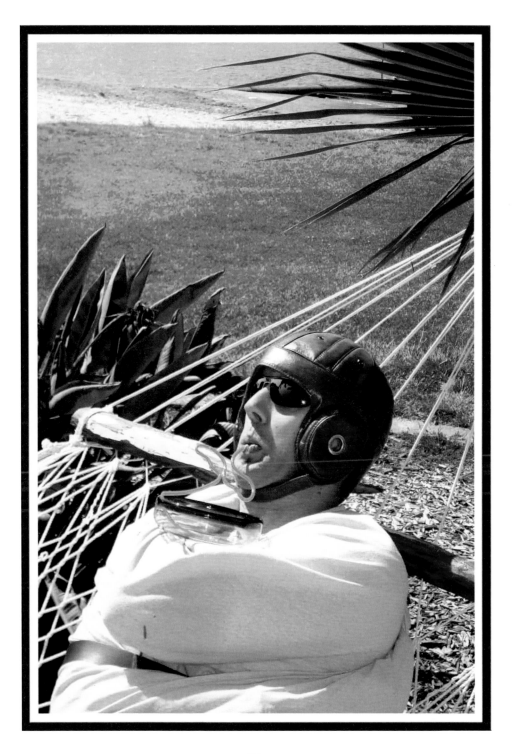

Straight Jacket in Paradise

If you are not right in the head or otherwise generally incapacitated, where do you want to be really? Shouldn't the mentally ill and people who have an extremely low tolerance for the rest of society be put on a cruise ship or an island instead of a padded room? What kind of shitty idea is that? How are padded walls supposed to help anxiety better than tide waves and beach sand? You can tie me up on an island of fools that's fine. Just give me sunlight and a massage and lots of the agave sauce. The only problem is that you have to keep shouting out for refills.

I couldn't get Nurse Yummy Tits (NE Erin) into the shot because she was working on another patient. Mentally unstable people of both sexes enjoy naughty nurses though. It's just a fact of life. She'll be in the movie though.

No editing was done to this photo.

Location: Fool's Island – Pacific Beach

Date Taken: Sometime in October 2009...

Photographers: Tracy & Diane

Model: This is me and I am flat-ass wasted drunk.

CLINICALLY FRUSTRATED

CHAPTER 1

Everything that you are about to read will make more sense keeping in mind that the author has been diagnosed with Tourette's syndrome. Additionally, people think that I am full-on bat-shit crazy. This is because they have no point of reference for judgment other than their own boring workaholic lives. Honestly I am only ¼ bat-shit crazy. First I will attempt to describe to you how it is that my higher brain functions work, strictly from my perspective. Then I shall give you what research data I have summarized.

I began this work as a therapy project for myself. At one point I remember having just over 100 pages and wondering if I shouldn't do something with it eventually.

TS is very similar to Parkinson's disease in that there really is no cure, treatment options are limited at best and it has a wide range of effects depending solely on the individual afflicted. It is about as funny as Alzheimer's disease, which is to say not very. Lately it has received a lot of unwarranted media attention by people claiming to have it and this does in fact piss me off since the afflicted person can easily determine who else might be a legitimate case.

During editing of this book I frequently had to correct problems of sentence structure and Dyslexia. This was never an actual symptom of mine and I once considered myself to be vocally eloquent, but rather these are side effects of the medications that I am on. It has taken some adjustment to get used to. At one point in time I took 5 weeks of medical leave just because I couldn't play nice anymore with the rest of the world. I never accrue vacation time or sick time and I even took bereavement time off when my fish died.

I will not even try to argue the point that my mind is completely demented by your standards. You will undoubtedly agree with this statement very quickly. Most of the time I could use an adult babysitter. If I am lucky, the publishing company will provide one when we do signings and appearances. It has to be a girl though and she has to be both hot and good at public relations.

THE WAY I SEE IT...

"...He said, you just can't win it. Everybody's in it for their own gain; you can't please 'em all." Joni Mitchell – *Free Man in Paris*

I cannot think of a more apropos phrase to explain my writings. The song goes on about the stress level of a record label executive. If memory serves me (I don't care to look up the facts on this, plus I think I am actually right), I believe it was written about David Geffen. This would be the same man who was rumored to have later done Carly Simon and made lots of cash so obviously life did get better for him after a few years despite the gay rumors. I thought he did Mariah Carey but I guess I'm wrong. I bet Mariah couldn't sing that high note during sex with my large member poking her diaphragm. I don't think that is a physical possibility.

Anyway...my point is that this is a phenomenal song that expresses the way many of us feel. We just want to walk away from it all. So how does this apply to me? Well, I get frustrated sometimes by the drop of a penny and the dropping of said penny is nothing at all to get mad at because there is little to no value in it. The more profound life stresses make me wish I could turn into the Incredible Hulk™ and destroy you all. You will notice that I like the Hulk because he doesn't lose.

My brain processes things at a much greater speed than the rate of what we will call a normal human brain. We will call it that because the majority of you do not have legitimate synaptic damage and/or increased processing capacity. The following is an arbitrary number not based on any clinical research, but let me guess for example that the mind of someone afflicted with TS draws conclusions perhaps 4 to 6 times faster.

Before you can even ask me where I want to eat I will have a list of my preferred options ready with an explanation of why I desire it at that given moment. It never fails. It is always this way. Furthermore, my lack of patience has earned me the nick name "Short Fuse". I don't like to make reservations for anything in advance and I expect everything to be perfect. I also expect that everybody I speak to should behave perfectly and give me the answers I want without hesitation. I don't have time for bull crap and I need a 3:00 pm nap. Currently, I really hate it when people don't call or write me back in a reasonable amount of time. If I... (The mentally unstable person) take the time out of my day to get in touch with you; you need to realize that you are important to me on some level and respond in kind. I can't be the only person alive who hates this.

I believe in my heart of hearts that this disorder is a punishment for something horrible I must have done in a former life. I hate it and it did lead to my divorce at least in part. You want to know why? It was because all the people who were close to me didn't think it was a legitimate problem, so I had no support, least of all from my wife or other family.

I have had to LEARN that I do not deserve preferential treatment. I have had to force myself to believe that I am not better than the rest of you. For years I truly thought that society did owe me something extra! I have tried but cannot shake this feeling. The only solace that I have from the bombardment of the world is my living space and bed which are a sanctuary. My beagle Daisy is my personal little angel. I am obsessively organized and lacking of clutter in general. Our home is considered to be my Holy Ground even though I am not holy.

TECHNICAL DEFINITION

Much of the information up until the next heading has been summarized from a report published by the Tourette Syndrome Association, Inc. in 1984. The article I found was entitled *A Physician's Guide to Diagnosis and Treatment of Tourette syndrome*. The paraphrased sections from that article are indented below. In short it reads:

> Tourette syndrome is a widely misunderstood genetically passed, neuro-behavioral disorder affecting as many as 1 in every 2500 people. T.S. is closely associated with the traits of obsession and compulsion as well as the disorders ADD and ADHD. T.S. however, is comprised of multiple parts and is usually not diagnosed as such unless the patient displays all the parts in some form or another.
>
> Symptoms generally develop in childhood in the form of transient or random tics. Nearly all children who are afflicted with the disorder will outgrow it completely around age 18. That being said, full-on adult cases are

rare. Usually if one of the components does stick around it is more likely to be a single chronic motor reflex tic.

Tourette syndrome does not mean swearing like a jack ass. Swearing can be one part of it and that part has its own name; Coprolalia. However, swearing without the other components does not mean you have TS. It just means you are a stupid bastard and you are taking up valuable oxygen that better people could use. In an unrelated story I hate "Goth" kids. Can we do without them? OK here come the symptoms, so strap in.

> Tics or twitches are predominant. They are involuntary, rapid, repetitive, and stereotyped movements of individual muscle groups. Sometimes the muscle groups are connected and sometimes they are not. Common tics include eye blinking, nose puckering, squinting, and winching of the neck shoulder and back muscles. Childhood tics may be bizarre, such as licking the palm or poking and pinching the genitals. Transient tics last only weeks or a few months and usually are not associated with specific behavioral problems. They are especially noticeable when a person's sensory perceptions become heightened as with excitement, happiness, anger or fatigue.

These are just a few examples. This stands true for me as nearly anything outside of emotional stability can begin a twitching episode.

> The presence of vocal or phonic tics is in addition to motor tics. Transient vocalizations are less common and include various throat sounds, humming, or other noises. As with all tic syndromes, boys are three to four times more often afflicted than girls. **Tourette Syndrome (TS)**, first described by Gilles de la Tourette, can be the most debilitating tic disorder, and is characterized by multiform,

frequently changing motor and phonic tics. Again, the prevailing diagnostic criteria include onset before the age of 21; recurrent, involuntary, rapid, **_purposeless_** motor movements affecting multiple muscle groups and one or more vocal tics. Some patients experience their tics as having a volitional component – that is to say they have an internal urge for motor discharge accompanied by psychological tension and anxiety likely because it is not easily controlled or stopped.

Simple motor tics: fast, darting, and meaningless.
Complex motor tics: slower, may appear purposeful
Simple vocal tics: meaningless sounds and noises.
Complex vocal tics: linguistically meaningful utterances such as words and phrases.
Often, but not always, vocal symptoms occur at points of linguistic transition, such as at the beginning of a sentence where there may be blocking or difficulties in the initiation of speech, or at phrase transitions. Coprolalia is the explosive utterance of foul or "dirty" words or more elaborate sexual and aggressive statements.

Coprolalia occurs in only a minority of TS patients being as little as 5%. It should be emphasized that a diagnosis of TS *does not require* that Coprolalia is present. My default war cry seems to be *"Fat Whore Bitch".* I'm not sure why.

All cases are slightly different. I have at one time or another experienced nearly all of the symptoms mentioned in the original report. The primary difference in my case was the onset of the disorder at about age 16. It has not ceased and in adult cases will likely never go away. On several occasions the muscle spasms have caused me a lot of internal injury. They can at times be violent. Therefore, I sought out medical help (which was not easy to find!) The treatment drug that I am on now is called Keppra. It is an anti-seizure drug, and was recommended as a best guess with the least amount of side effects. It helps but nothing stops the tics. I also have some wonderful prescription level anxiety medicine, which works by knocking me cold on my ass for 14 hours.

FÜCKIN

Forced Unlawful Carnal Knowledge: I'm pretty sure someone made that up but at least it works. Just so you know my mother and my girlfriend recently did some etymology research on this word because my mom just hates it. The best they can do is trace it back to about 1500 A.D. Germanic and Scandinavian cultures. The best of the many usages I have found is that when peoples of the community would catch an adulterer they would put them in the stocks (the actual wooded neck and arm holders) and burned into the wood above their heads would be the word "fuckin" (yes, without the g at the end). Now since it is rather hard to trace and because of their accents I am suggesting that they phonetically pronounced it as (foo-kin) hence my use of the letter Ü. That's just a guess though. Some English scholar probably civilized it later and it became a formal verb.

TRIGGERS

In context, a trigger is something that makes a person either very happy or very angry. It applies to many different neurological disorders. You have them too even if you are normal. It's just a topic that gets you fired up. We also like to call it passion. One could safely assume that everything that I write about is pretty much a trigger for me, but in particular we have found that my really hot buttons include the following:

- Driving Slowly and People Not Paying Attention
- Math and Sales Metrics
- Telephones in General
- Obesity
- Homosexuality
- Screaming Children
- Commercials
- Fluorescent Lighting
- Sudden Loud Noises (alarm clocks, car horns...)

Side effects of the drugs that I have noticed include:
- Slurred and Stuttered Speech
- Writing Difficulties and Minor Dyslexia
- Loss of Congruent Sleep Time
- Lack of Focus
- Increased Verbal Outbreaks
- Symptomatic Related Depression

TICS

As a subject that I have some authority on, tics or twitching of the neck, shoulders, face and other parts of the body are terribly disturbing. They are annoying and disfiguring always at a time when someone you care about seems to be watching. While they can be funny to observe, a good rule of thumb is to never upset a person with this condition if you are aware that it visually exists.

Now I am one of the better natured beings on the planet and I have been fortunate not to really cut off anybody's head when I was laughed at, but I certainly wanted to. In fact the ridicule has set a rather disturbing and violent thought pattern in my mind that remains today. If a solution to whatever I am facing does not present itself in a timely manner, I begin to daydream about violence.

What should you do if you know somebody with this apparent twitching condition called Chronic Motor Tics? Certainly do not ridicule them and certainly do not continue to recommend that they see a doctor. First of all you should get out of their way and let them be alone for a while. If that is not an option then just start giving them anything they want. They will reciprocate with kindness, and although the tic may not stop right away the gestures you're making will be appreciated. When you are not with this person next, try to think of what has changed in your lives or relationships together. Did they not get enough fresh air? Do they not handle large crowds well? Are you not paying enough attention to this person? They tend to need a lot of it. If it is your spouse, is there a lack of sex or desire to constantly touch? People with tics are highly sensitive and physical, so I'm sure that it is not for their lack of trying. Whatever it is, if the tic has developed since you met the person and was not always there, then something has changed and it is your responsibility to figure it out. Let me give you a clue, if you really know how to listen they will tell you every few minutes. You're probably just tired of hearing it and don't want to recognize what it is. Give them what they want or get out of their lives if you cannot.

PSYCHOLOGISTS

Contrary to what you may have thought, those with tics are extremely proud and strong willed people. If we understand what our trigger points are then all we have to do is avoid them. There is nothing that anyone else can help us with.

The previous section on tics is what brings me to tell you about my views on psychology and mental health institutions. As I understand it, some astounding fraction of the population has at one time or another in their lives been to see a psychiatrist or counselor. It is my opinion that many people who go to one just desire something they cannot have.

Think about what you want for a moment. Custody of your children? Large denomination cash? Proper sentence structure? This sure ain't it. It may be love, or an old toy, or a pet. I'm telling you that the only thing you can do to help if it is within your power is to just give it to 'em man! End the pain. End the suffering. I want to go to an institution every day because I have to deal with the reality of being middle class. There in the home they would take care of me, and comfort me, and somebody else would wipe my ass for me. If they wanted to pretend to cure me, all they would have to give me would be good food, hot water, sunshine and a daily back massage. That's all! End of story! I'm cured! Halleluiah and praise be to the saints!

DREAMS

Dreams are powerful things that we do not yet understand. I believe that the unpredictability of mine may be in part to the daily physical and ensuing mental torture that I endure.

I equate my personal dreams to being in a state of dementia. That for a living person is of course a terrible thing. Who is to really say if they are cognoscente of being awake? I realize that I can be a jerk but in all sincerity my heart goes out to these people to whom I can relate. I imagine Alzheimer's patients could best be described as living in a constant state of Dementia. Some Foundation that deals with these disorders will likely be willed all of my cash when I die. That should be just about $17.50.

When I describe my dreams I usually cannot find the words to accurately relate what happens inside of them. They are sometimes lucid, often euphoric and every time vivid. I cannot stand up immediately as I am left with a sense of vertigo. The funny thing is that during maybe 27 nights out of the month the substance of my dreams are better than that of real life. Is it any wonder that I prefer a nap at 3 o'clock pm?

Dreams unquestionably deserve to be discussed. You can in no way convince me that dreams do not mean anything. The meaning may be misconstrued by our conscience mind or lost in intuitive translation as it were; but they damn sure mean something to me. I make it a point to tell all of my friends and acquaintances, no matter how awkward it seems at the time, exactly what role they played in the dream.

I wonder if dreaming isn't akin to sending yourself to the astral plane. Your mind is free to wander and encounter any number of things. I see people all the time whom I know in real life but who are acting out of character thus alerting some innate sense of mine that I am actually asleep. This is arguably a necessary step in determining lucid dreaming: the ability to control some aspects of the dream realm.

At sunrise (since I refuse to use an alarm clock) I wake up and have to lie in bed for at least 30 minutes, reeling in the fact that my dream was so realistic that I feel lost. Furthermore, it impairs my judgment and temperament for the better part of the following 2 hours.

So I have had dreams about becoming quite powerful in many facets and I very often gain extraordinary power. I have a few recurring nightmares. One is about being in school for eternity and the other is about having "dead air" while on the radio. Not just a few seconds, but like 4 minutes worth! That one makes me sweat every time.

I really dislike dreams about my ex-wife. I don't hurt her of course, just her fat Porky Pig™ friend. Actually, it was me and Clint Eastwood in a gun fight against "the pig" and 8 other losers. Needless to say I mopped the floor with the guys he didn't kill.

In my dreams I have a full range of telekinetic power. I crush vehicles with my mind and then throw them great distances. I can light things on fire and generally enjoy doing so. I am in love with the current wave of super hero / villain movies that have come out in the last 5 years because that is the world I live in when I am asleep. *Hancock* rose to the top of my list pretty quickly. You can imagine why. Random destruction, all day long……….

In one of my all time favorite dreams, I not only have the ability to fly (which many of you can relate to) but I have beautiful wings with an enormous span and I use my abilities to follow girls around. I perch in a tree sometimes and wait for them to get naked, because the act of watching someone get naked is usually better than the sum of what you see when they are fully in that state.

The list goes on and on about ridiculous dreams that I have. Every morning I could catalogue a new one for you that could…at best be put into the format of a collegiate film school project.

RECAP

I am sorry for this but you don't play on my level. I like things that go fast and I make snap decisions. I don't have the patience to work in one location and I can't sit still. I crave sunlight like Birdman™. I don't have regrets. I have made mistakes that I have turned into a life lesson. My body, while the upper half is studly, is also habitually sore. I communicate better with animals than I do with people.   I was blessed with a giant cock.

For editing purposes I gave the rough draft book to 3 people to look over. The point was mainly to tell me if it was not understandable since I can be long-winded. I was told by one of the women that it sounds like this whole chapter was about how awesome I thought I was. She assumed the rest of the book would come across that way also. I have to address that and also say thank you. It does kind of come off that way; however I must not be that awesome because otherwise I wouldn't be frustrated and people would just do the things I suggest to them without making a big stink. They would just have the realization that they were in the presence of human mental greatness. If they want to be a better person they would take my lessons to heart. To make an analogy, it would be like your friend asking you whom they should date, but then they don't ever listen to you and continue to have shitty relationships. I hope that clears it up.

The point of this whole chapter was to get you to realize that the disorder is more prevalent than you think. I would bet that every reader could pick out at least one acquaintance that they have made in their lifetime that has exhibited some of these symptoms. Maybe they didn't have full blown TS. Perhaps they just had a chronic blinking tic. That one is common but it's no less frustrating for the victim. So now that you know I implore you to be kind and give that person just a little extra attention. They will love you for it.

I couldn't have written this particular book if I didn't know something about the subject and there wasn't an audience to learn about my life and my ways so truly I could not have done it without you. Let's move on to the next chapter shall we?

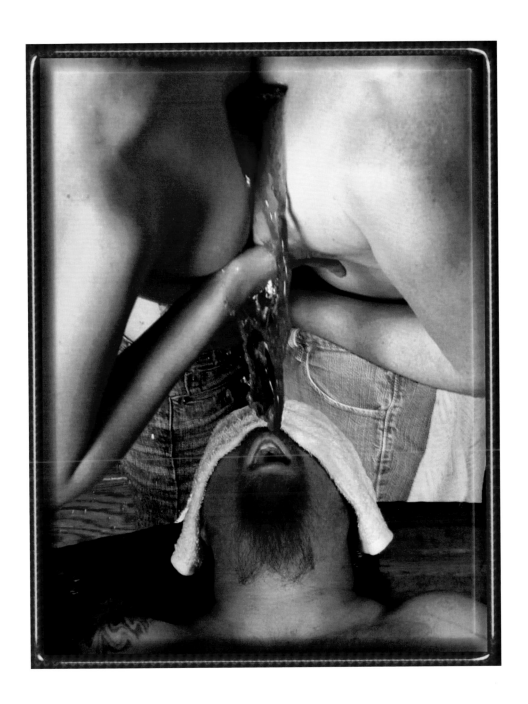

Body Shots

Body Shots is a classic picture and it's my idea so I fully expect royalties from anyone selling this type of thing as a service even if you only use one girl with gi-normous boobs. I thought of that too but I had time and money constraints. I now know why no one else has attempted it before. It took way too much work to actually pull this off and I needed way more than just my two hands. The angles were nearly impossible to get right. We tried several things before getting the whisky barrel and a big ladder. A big thank you goes out to the models.

The message here is that taking a shot from someone's hand or licking their arm or shoulder is ludicrous. The whole point of the body shot is to be sucking on a more desirable part of their body anyway. Full-on body shots from the reservoir between the breasts should be allowed in public bars. Who cares about the price? Raise it up. Don't you think those women should be compensated who put up with that kind of behavior? I do. I'm just saying it should be done, that's all. Beating around the bush is a waste of time and it doesn't please the rest of the crowd either. Oh yeah, the patron definitely gets to lick the girls for clean up. We used a towel for this one to protect his eyes and his identity. He did complain the whole time about the towel!

Photography   Arnold Coleman
Lighting   Hawksdream Photography
Model agent   Denver, CO

Concept   Parrish Douglas
Photo Editing

GENERAL GRIPES, BITCHES, PUBLIC OPINION & RUMORS

CHAPTER II

This chapter is included solely for the purpose of inciting riots and inter-office chatter. The views expressed in this chapter are not necessarily the opinions of my agent or any member of the publishing or distributing companies. They are my opinions alone. Any similar opinions expressed by anyone you know are purely coincidental.

This chapter is also completely random, much like the way I speak and act in real life. I suggest against trying to rationally follow my train of thought. You might hurt yourself.

Furthermore, the grammar in this section in positively atrocious. I am not going to change it however. I did make fair warning in the Foreword to my new literary style, which is plenty full of apostrophes and hyphenations and assorted verbiage.

I do use the term "Gay" a lot here but that is addressed in the Sex chapter just so you know. Don't get your panties in a wad.

13 RANDOM THOUGHTS

1) **Theme Park** - There needs to be one constructed for adults called "Self-Indulgent Pleasure Land". Put it in Tennessee where that stuff is legal. It should include such attractions as a beer slide with a beer pool at the bottom. Booby-Land, where you can go to take a nap after the beer pool. A huge racecar track and separate demolition derby. There would be a fighting equipment arena with large gloves, sumo suits and padded lances with platforms above mud. It needs a full on obstacle course and a wrestling ring. Gambling allowed on everything. Paintball guns issued at the door. Luxury Castle, where you can get a massage or sit in a hot tub and watch a giant TV. There would be an S & M Dungeon where you get to either watch or sign up for the action. A shooting and archery range with explosives behind the targets. Bungee cords, speed bumper boats, human cannons and the Jell-O gelatin moonwalk. Zip-lines between the attractions and finally the biggest all inclusive open bar and buffet of all time with a bed to crash in or you can stumble back to Booby-land.

2) **Field Testing** - Scientists should develop something like a truth strip that resembles a PH testing strip for a pool or spa. The difference being that you would dip this into somebody's beverage at the table or bar. It could turn colors to tell you if they are lying. It would help considerably when dating. They could take it one step further and just make Chemistry / Compatibility test kits and that could be the new thing to do at the bars. Oh yeah, we need a finger pricker for communicable diseases also.

3)   <u>**Fat**</u> – There is an old cruise ship joke about the showers being too small and how it's easier to soap up the wall first and then just spin around. Yes they are small but if your fat touches the wall it's not the showers fuckin' fault. I fit in there just fine. Be honest with yourself.   Too many people wrongly hold themselves in high regard. You weren't meant to be the size of an SUV. The sight of a 350lb+ human being makes me physically nauseous. Tank-ass is a serious problem in this country. Don't take a plate of bacon on the cruise ship just 'cause it's free! You people need some damn help. Tell your family "I'm moving in and you're gonna help me. You now have the right to punch me." Next, quit your job. You can't fuckin' work effectively anyway. After you're in shape you won't want that same old job.   Then you rally all the money you can and go down to the clinic and just *get that fatty shit sucked out of you.* You'll be plenty strong from carrying all that baggage around. Your body however will be used to producing toxins and storing fat so you still have to not eat pig bacon.   There you go. I have fixed your life for you.   You're welcome and I thank you for not making me projectile vomit anymore. Muffin tops; I want to kill you. Disney™ could not have made a better statement than in whole movie **WALL•E**™. Bravo!

<u>Statement of Humility:</u> I am shortly going to be handicapped myself. My joints are going bad at an accelerated rate so I won't be able to work out and may have seriously have to consider liposuction. I want it to be known that I am fully aware of my own hypocrisy on this subject. It is not right to support the discrimination or ridicule of these persons as in my life many of the nicest people I have met have had these disabilities. The statements contained within are intended to encourage realization and the path to improvement. We should not make fun of these people but rather we should try to help them. Sometimes help starts by getting out of the house and getting some honest opinions. Be a friend when they need one or a counselor or support mechanism.   We should try to love all people for their true nature and being. If you witness me being

cruel, I invite you to correct me. The TS does make me occasionally lose it when you get in my way.

4) **Music Styles** - Country is not all bad, and I want to state this for the record. It just takes some getting used to. Liking country music is a learned behavior much like learning to drive fast or swim underwater. At first it seems a little uncomfortable but then you get used to it. At the very least, almost all of the artists can play their instruments very well. It takes a lot of hard work and years of practice and self-sacrifice to be able to rip scales in every key like they do.

Rap Music is one of the biggest verbal contradictions in the entire English language. There's rarely an original tune without any tracks dubbed in from an older song. Rap and its spin off sister "hip hop" are for losers and anyone that likes either of the two is simply a fudge-packer. I have no use for you. OK, not really but truly good songs in this genre (eek, I hate calling it that) are few and far between.

Now then, extremely hard rock or metal rock is just embarrassing, and power ballads by any band should be outlawed. They serve no other point than to annoy the super-intelligent. Therefore anyone who likes hard rock should be condemned to life as a virtual slave until such time as they see the error of their ways. In fact, most of them are mindless zombies even without their knowledge. Too drugged out to know the difference between real life and a having fun by getting high. There are a few exceptions like those who were given money, made a wise investment, or work at a radio station. For the most part though, their appearance and attitudes are the very things that condemn them to be underlings in society.

POWER BALLADS *SUCK* and IF YOU LIKE POWER BALLADS THAN *YOU SUCK* TOO!

5) **Daytime TV Talk Shows** - are completely pointless and spineless from a man's point of view. Seriously, you can't find anything better to do? Talking about your problems on national television doesn't solve anything. I say put the contestants in a ring and let them have brutal and physically demanding matches. I don't care. It will increase ratings. The people who come on talk shows are pretty much fucked up beyond the chance for help anyway, so the networks might as well give them the personal satisfaction of allowing them to fulfill their dream of beating the pulp out of their most hated enemy in a venue that will not wind them up in jail. There just is no better fight than one spawned by a cheating spouse. I would even go so far as to say make it a handicapped match wherein the person who did the cheating, or even the person they cheated with has their ankles cuffed so that they must remain on a lower level than the innocent party. If they still manage to be victorious by luck or by superior fighting skill than I guess someone will get it through their heads that it's time to move on won't they?

6) **Scotches** - Why in the hell do people keep reading material in their restrooms? I can understand that you just had a major bowel movement and that it took a lot of energy out of you, but if that is the case shouldn't you just put your head down for a minute or make a loud noise of relief. Do you really need to read something to take your mind off the unpleasant task of cleaning yourself? Why in the hell do most people apparently not clean themselves totally after having a movement? When did having bacon strips or skid marks become acceptable? If I was a woman and I saw that in my partner's drawers I would absolutely never see him again. Not an arguable point here. If the circumstance arises that you have an accident or regularly break wind to the affect that you splatter and think it's funny, then you need to keep a spare pair of shorts in the glove box of your car and you damn sure should just throw the old ones away!

7) Luggage - Immigrants pack entirely too much damn luggage. Now having worked at an international airport for some time I feel that I have the right to say "Screw you guys!" I don't know what the reason behind packing a two hundred pound tweed *"maleta"* is, but I can tell you that it doesn't bode well with the ramp agents. Neither does placing 7 or 8 fragile stickers on it. I will tell you honestly right now that we say "fragile my ass" and then power bomb your bag. We punch them, we hit them with other bags, we hold distance throwing contests giving extra points for however many wheels we break off, and my favorite, if you are a teenage girl with a cute name and pink luggage we will take your panties out and put them in our lockers. So don't pack canned foods, and stop sending liquor bottles. Buy it when you get there. Don't send dead chickens or your children in luggage, we will hurt them. And don't cry to us when we do.

8) Telephone Customer Service - If there is one thing that universally everyone in the world hates, it's the damn automated answering systems that all major corporations have now. Dear Lord Christ, I beseech you now to please damn these mother-fucking things straight to hell. In their defense I can understand that they don't want to take calls from the 20 million losers who can't figure out how to work a DVD for example. That is what the system was developed for, to filter out the losers and to eliminate one more person's good job from the potential field of opportunity. But now it has gotten out of control in epic proportions. The IRS is the worst. Everyone in the country is referred to one number. But anyway, I'm all about offering solutions and I really do like to speak with a human on the phone. It just makes one feel not quite so inconsequential.

Any company wishing to make a bold statement about how much they care for their customers should rehire one or two telephone support personnel who are born ENGLISH speaking AMERICANS located, working and living in AMERICA! These positions should be glorified as something that requires a lot of patience and great communications skills. It should carry with it a glorious salary as well like say $60,000 to start with anti-frustration bonuses on top of that. Would you like to speak to a helpful, happy person who makes $60,000+ a year on the phone? I would, and I would also gladly give the company who employed that person my business for life.

9)   Insects - Fuck I hate a lot of bugs. Only because they act irrationally, move erratically and get in your face. I thought I covered this already but I can't find it. As far as I can tell, we only need about 8 kinds of bugs on the whole planet. We can biologically kill off all the rest and that will be just fine, especially crickets and mosquitoes! Then we'll genetically mass produce the good kinds. These being: ladybugs, lightning-bugs, rollie-pollie-bugs, honey bees, regular ants, really pretty butterflies, daddy long legs spiders and earthworms. That's all we need! Think about the brilliance of it. All the nasty annoying things like flies and moths would be gone and the world would be filled with lightning bugs. That's a warm and fuzzy feeling right there.

10)   Small Children - should not be allowed at adventure parks like Disneyland, in any shopping mall, or at any entertainment mediums such as concerts or movie theaters. I'm talking small children here that don't even understand a whole lot of English or any other language. Less than 2 years old. Don't fool yourself. They don't have the patience and neither do I to listen to their screaming. What are they doing exactly? Enjoying hot, overcrowded spaces? They slow you down *AND* they don't know what's going on anyway so what is the point? You are into self-torture perhaps? I scream back and thankfully people grab their kids and run away. Woe is the parent who tries to get in a yelling match with me. You don't even know loud.

11)   Holiday Shopping - Department stores that hold their' holiday sales 3 months in advance of the event should be burned. Yes, I'm speaking of arson. I don't want to see Valentine's Day crap the day after Christmas. I DON'T WANT TO SEE IT! I really don't care about up selling or how much revenue they can drive by staging the product early either. It just looks stupid and 90% of all shoppers say it's ridiculous. Please boycott any holiday products until 2 weeks before the event. Better yet, put something in your cart and then give it to the cashier and tell that person you don't want it anymore because you're just not in the mood for Easter in late February.

12) <u>**Radio**</u> - Morning shows can be terribly annoying. Most of the people are not entertainers to begin with. How do these pig fuckers get their jobs? They didn't go to school for it. I did go to school just for that and I can tell you there are almost no people on the air today with an actual damn broadcasting degree. Especially to you Program Directors I say WTF? None of you accept phone calls yet you are supposed to be professionals at communicating. "I'm too busy" is just an excuse for "I suck at my job" or I'm busy sucking my boss right now and can't take your call. I will also be honest and tell you I have thought about shooting bad DJ's from 400 yards out. I practice with HALO.

You don't have to have a degree that's fine, however you really need to get a grasp on things and fire some people. It's not uncommon to also have teams (that suck), which have gotten away with sucking for like 12 years! Adult Contemporary formats are the worst for this. On top of that you have the fact that normal humans don't act all happy and fun until at least 10:00 when their shows are usually over. Hear me out... Put me back on the air. Not every day but certainly once in a while, let me bitch and complain and sip my coffee in front of the microphone. I'll take calls from people who say their bones are creaking and they got in a wreck on the way to work and they'd like to just hear their favorite song so they could turn it up really loud and forget about the world for 3 min 41 sec. I am telling you there is a huge market for this kind of morning show. Nobody likes happiness at 7 am deep down in their soul. I don't buy it.

One more thing; this whole bullshit that every station is doing about "breaking the rules" and "playing whatever they want", that is a fucking retarded **BOLDFACE LIE**. You want to break the rules? Play the Four Fucking Tops on a Country station. Play the Jim Brickman song Valentine on a damn Alternative station. Most people have a mix of shit in their iPods now anyway. You're breaking the rules about as much as my intestine breaks down corn. Fuckers.

13) <u>**Coughing**</u> - What is it that people don't understand about the physical act of coughing? I want my Mother to know this is directly aimed at her (with love). A person has 2 fucking pipes in their throat! An air pipe and a food pipe. When food OR LIQUID goes down the air pipe you cough. You know why? Because your lungs are supposed to be DRY! It is you body's natural reaction to force the shit out of the wind pipe...ergo...taking a drink of water WILL NOT HELP YOU!!!!!!! Don't tell other people to put more water down an already bad pipe, plus you can't even consciously do that! How do you knowingly swallow water into your lungs? You put water into your stomach, which doesn't help the problem. Just cough it up, baby. That's what you gotta do.

MORE ON MUSIC

As music is a big part of all of our lives, don't you think that we should be more respectful and diligent about giving credit where credit is due? Yeah, young POP star vocalists sell records and that's fine; someone has to. They are hot and I would screw them, sure. What I'm saying is that the monetary split needs to be right down the middle. Let's say for example that on a Jessica Simpson CD there were a total of 6 full time professional musicians and 3 full time studio techs. Oh, there were also 2 songwriters, because she is actually not a musician at all and poetry lyrics only count for $1/4^{th}$ of an actual song composition. With her vocals that makes a total of 12 people involved with the sound engineering of the project. She can make all the money she wants on the side by selling her image, but I strongly disapprove of anyone making more than their fare share on the sales of the CD just because they are a prima donna vocalist.

You couldn't make shit without the studio people and you damn well know it. In this scenario Jessica Simpson should make only $1/12^{th}$ of the royalties after the record company takes out all of their fees. Would she be independently wealthy if she didn't take on some other task? Probably not.

This is why we like bands. The term band implies that everyone collaborated and is getting equal credit. Bands kick ass, but when you have problems then just let it die. Don't add new members...let it die or rename the group with "version 2" on the end. Remember, POP stars = bad. Studio guys = good.

MORE ON TELEVISION

First off, why can't you dick-bags learn to engineer the fucking sound volume on a commercial correctly? I know how to do this. I am a sound engineer by trade. Everyone on planet earth (including you) hates to have to turn down the TV when the commercials come on. I personally just mute the thing 'cause most of them are gay anyway. Only Superbowl commercials should be louder and you also know damn well that their volume can be pumped up on the back end at the broadcast studio just before it goes on the air. I actually had a Superbowl etiquette conversation with my nephew Ryan when he was 8 years old. *Fix the problem bitches!*

Now for programming: All television programs and movies should fall into one of my four categories. These are:

C - Children's
L - Lame Shows for Lame People
A - Adult in nature
P - Pornographic

A - Adult in Nature rating is to include all things like crime, language, innuendo and comedies that pass out of the Lame Shows category. In order for a comedy or daytime drama not to earn the Lame rating there must be some exposed boobies with nipple shown during every scene where two people sleep together. There is not one woman in the world who takes the sheets with them when they go to the kitchen or when they sit up to talk about something. No, just...no. Furthermore a show will not automatically get the Pornographic rating just for showing boobies; it must be a hardcore program. The cable show <u>Sex in the City</u> for example must be made to have real sex in it or risk being publicly labeled Lame. Come on, it's supposed to have sex!

Now here is an example of the Lame category; Angela Lansbury, although a very creative soul, is also a misguided and sick person. Her character of Jessica on *Murder She Wrote* would not only have been beaten senseless, shot, stabbed, gang raped and humiliated but filled internally with rocks and sank to the bottom of the river for meddling in the affairs of the criminal world. At least if I were a criminal I can say that I would have killed her, and in the pilot episode might I add. The premise for the show is so weak that I originally thought she must have given one hell of a blowjob to the network people but I would be wrong. My close friend tells me that she was the Executive Producer which really means Financier. Can't they just say that? Don't lie to us. It is what it is.

CHILDREN'S TV PROGRAMMING

Above all else under this heading it is important to note that the 1980's *Transformers, GI Joe, Thundercats* and *He-Man* were some of the best children's shows that were ever produced. Sure it had an occasional bad rendering and they got the character names wrong but by their own admission they were cranking these episodes out by hand, unlike today where computers give the assist. Recently the episodic drama *Dragonball Z* has achieved worldwide justified fame. The animation is not bad at all while still retaining a healthy sense of action and urgency. The Japanese do however have a fancy for story lines that go on forever. I heard it was produced in 1985!

I HATE (and I'm not alone) watching anything, TV or film, in which a child or a stupid cat saves the world. I can't express in writing how much I hate this. It makes me want to throw things at the walls. It just doesn't happen people. It's stupid by make-believe standards! What's the attraction here? Wouldn't you rather fantasize about beating the hell out of your incompetent boss or your abusive boyfriend or something? Winning the lottery? Something? Judges?

The fact is that children can't save their missing P.O.W. fathers from Korea, and they can't foil master criminal schemes, and they can't catch robbers or bad guys. They certainly lack the physical strength necessary to do these stunts and they would be killed or at least tied up and beaten. Even large dogs or cats that try this would definitely be killed and probably eaten for lunch. Hypothetically speaking, if I were a criminal in the middle of committing a large crime to make me very wealthy and all that stood in my way was a filthy slobbery animal, child, or full grown adult for that matter, they would find themselves holding hands with the previously mentioned "Jessica" at the bottom of a very cold deep river or lake. Criminals are mean! That's why they're criminals!

Here's another thing. Saturday morning children's programming has gone straight to hell with very few exceptions. What happened to learning from the masters? Chuck Jones, Hanna / Barbara and the like. The amount of new animation that is produced for daily shows is mostly crap. This would be insufferable as a child to me. Especially the shows that aren't even cartoons! The last thing I wanted to see on Saturday morning was a real person on my TV. You know what would have happened to the Power Rangers if I was the bad guy? Knife to the heart! Even the girls!

To make it easier on myself so that I don't have a brain aneurism, here is an example list of intolerable programming. There is more, but this will give you an idea of what not to watch. If I planned on having children, there would be no way in the fiery fires of hell that they would watch these shows. I have also expressed my opinions to my brother who has kids. The list:

- Any gay ass live action show with any resemblance to the Power Rangers.
- Big Fucker Barney and his butt plugging pals with televisions in their stomachs.
- Saved by the Bastard-Ass Bell
- That piece of crap show (Full House) with that putrid, broom in his ass, skinny faggot guy that did the funny video shows. **
- That bitch Erkle show.

In short if it's not Muppets or a cartoon w/ more than 3 frames per second, it's crap. Even in reruns the Muppet Show was one of the best-produced television shows ever! Generally acceptable cartoons will have a heavy regiment of super-heroes and war.

**As a side note I have nothing against the twin girls personally and I should like to have wild sex with both of them in a vat of fruit cocktail with light sauce. The show wasn't their faults'. They were cute. They just did what the adults told them to do.

Last and least is Reality TV. I'm too busy living my own damn life to worry about some MTV Road Rash crap and _YOU_ should be too busy also! What would be entertaining in this genre (if you can call it that) would be a World's Strongest Gay Man competition or something functional like a Rubberneckers Car Crash show for the people who feel they have to slow down to look at everything. I personally hate you people. Just crash your own fuckin' car in ditch and look at that for a while. Get off my road!

THE MOVIES

Let it be known that absolutely NO movie should get a 5 star or 2 thumbs up rating without the following: **_FULL FRONTAL NUDITY and EXPLOSIONS!_**

I have always had a fascination with the boobs and the element of fire. They translate into so many aspects of my life. They nurture a group of base feelings and emotions. Passion, energy, growth; things that make you feel alive. That's why they are necessary to a good, believable film.

Things that do not make a good film would include pompous actors. There are people in Hollywood that are horrible. I'm sure that they are very personable, wonderful human beings to meet, however they are not believable in any role they take on other than that of a normal loser with an average job and a hideously ugly mate. They should not attempt to portray pilots, spies, congressman, or lawyers. I have been told by several of my friends who are actors that listing names in my book would surely be an act of professional suicide if I intended to enter into the field myself. I thought about it but decided I didn't care since I have pushed the envelope with everything else. You, the reader would not respect me at all if I didn't tell you. We (the working class ugly people) greatly outnumber them. Revenge of the Nerds is awesome!!! Here we go...

Currently Tom Cruise and Justin Timberlake are at the top of my list. Brad Pitt surprisingly worked his way off that list after 7 Years in Tibet. There is also one other person whose initials are A.K. He is a turd swallowing circus performer at best. I can't write his name here because I made a personal vow never to speak it again and he makes me vomit. He has also ruined many wonderful actresses for me so I hate him on a personal level too. Oh yeah, I also dislike all of the Sheens'. All of the people in this paragraph look too good, and never have bad teeth or hair. This is not real life and it doesn't make them believable in their roles. Any man who likes any part of their acting has some hidden issues that they need to explore with a professional counselor. I don't hate many actresses but I really don't like Meryl Streep. She scares me a little in a manly way.

In addition, I would like to not see ANY actor or actress in more than 3 major headlining roles EVER, with little exception. The only one being that if they have done their 3 films and would then like to show some skin for publicity's sake, then that would be acceptable. Then even no more than 1 additional film that would require the full fledged super-star to include a full frontal shot and possibly penetration. Many people just get tired of seeing their faces again and again and we want new blood. Make way for other people who would like to fulfill their dreams of acting but are closed out of the industry. Casting Directors need to do a lot more raw talent scouting in places other than their back yards.

Just two more small notes on this subject to use as examples: This is movie frustration → Independence Day – The scene right after the aliens had fired the big weapon on Los Angeles. Mom, kid and dog are running for shelter in the tunnel and she happens to find an open maintenance closet. Did you see all the other people in that tunnel? Don't you think they would be packing it into that closet with her? Don't you think that dog's ass would be burnt? Frankly, I think so. These people are desperate. I would have punched her in the face and thrown her out myself, purely as an instinctual reaction. There would have been no pre-meditated thought.

This is sweet movie justice → The *Lost World - Jurassic Park* The scene where the T-Rex is in San Diego in someone's back yard and he eats the family dog. Folk's, I went to the premiere of that movie in a 500-seat theater, and when that happened I was cheering. *People were booing at me!* This is a large hungry dinosaur. If the dog didn't die I was ready to walk out. All the kids were crying but that's life. Too bad they didn't show it. I wonder if it's in the director's cut?

SPORTS

Major league sports players should have to first gain residency in whatever town they decide to make a deal with. If the team players all hail from within the cities' limits, it will help to build a better sense of community, as well as give more opportunity to young players who would not otherwise get a chance.

In addition, it pisses me off that the salary cap for professional sports players is not more like $300,000 or so with full lifetime medical and a shorter term for retirement pay. The guys that need to be payed more money are the support personnel who work for the airlines, construction workers, nurses, store clerks, stockmen and other people who give us help and do the jobs that make our lives more comfortable. If they really love to play and be in the spotlight, they'll still do it. If not, fuck 'em. Let's use robots with nerds as the drivers. That would be awesome if they had digital face pictures of nerds on the players with really huge robotic bodies. If you are a sports player reading this right now, don't cry. It only makes you look like more of a pussy.

I have to say this because it bothers me so much. *STOP RUNNING THE FOOTBALL UP THE FUCKING MIDDLE!!!!! WHO CAME UP WITH THAT DUMB ASS PLAY? NEVER EVER RUN THE FOOTBALL UP THE FUCKING MIDDLE YOU DOUCHE BAG!!!!!* It doesn't work. In what world (exactly) do you think that it works? In this world it maybe flies one out of 1,000 times. Is that good?

OK, there are also too many fowls in professional sports. Basketball for example is a sport filled with whiners. What the fuck is a travelling call? Some shit like you can't take more than 2 steps without bouncing the ball? Gay! And then you're not allowed to punch the ball out of somebody's hands. Also Gay! I play tackle basketball and baseball, not very often of course because I'm rather skinny and it hurts. I propose a new additive for professional teams to make things more interesting; special rules that make personal injury the only allowable foul. This will test the true competitive nature and abilities of our athletes. You could go so far as to include a mandatory overtime with no rules for the Super Bowl, Stanley Cup and all that jazz. Showmanship on the field would be encouraged. No time outs. No flags for fags. If after you factor in all those things and people still want to roid-up and die early then let 'em. We need to push the boundaries of evolution.

Ooo! One more thing: professional **WRESTLING**! Yeah baby! I watch this stuff because I am simply amazed at how large a person can grow their muscles. I personally have tried everything on the planet <u>except</u> for anabolic steroids and Human Growth Hormone. I know what I'm talking about when I say people don't grow that large on their own. Now the height you can't induce and Mother Nature does make us all slightly different so you technically could have been a fat kid that worked out, but damn!

I want to be Batista or Khali for a day just so I could throw ice cream at people in suits. Then I'd look at 'em and say "What?" A lot of people believe that it is a totally fake sport. I don't personally care because they entertain me. I would caution the naysayers though to try some of that shit and see if it doesn't break you in half. I have lots of bad body parts including my back. I see a power-bomb go down...I would stop breathing and so would you. Bottom line; don't call wrestling fake or you are also not only a pussy, but an armchair warrior pussy. Thank you.

TURNING OLD

Talking about my broken parts leads me into this. I think I have said this a few times, so I am already going senile or I am really stressed out over this point. Old people, when they lose their facilities have no business trying to be in a young persons' world. *This goes for me too when I get there.* Just don't even try to buy anything with a microchip if you have to ask a question about it.

And stop freakin' driving already! Use the old people trams to go to the technology stores. Store associates that have to answer questions are severely underpaid. These places should designate and pay handsomely for someone to deal with the questions of old people. I did this job (not by choice but because I needed the money) for a while at several locations so I know how frustrating they can be.

One ridiculous example of my point is the story of an old lady that I was forced to help once with an answering machine. It seems that she was all pissed off that the manufacturer had installed a man's voice (electronic message) from the factory and she couldn't do anything about it. Of course when I asked her if she read the directions she said yes. She even used the word "asinine" toward me when describing the product. At that point I was obligated to make her look like a dirty "culo". (That's slang for ass-hole in Spanish). She was dense. I spoke down to her for 40 minutes and did 3 product demonstrations, which included letting her push the buttons. It finally sunk in when I recorded a message for her in a sarcastic girly voice that said, "Hi, I can't follow instructions and I need help to wipe my ass." Followed with, "Think you can get it now?"

I was consequently fired but she'll never forget that _rude_ salesman that made her feel like a three-year-old child.

JUST READ THE GOD-DAMMED DIRECTIONS. IF YOU CAN'T GET IT, READ THEM AGAIN OR TAKE IT BACK. DON'T SAY ONE STUPID WORD ABOUT GETTING HELP.

And *MICROSOFT* / ALL computer manufacturers – stop putting crap on the machines straight out of the factories! Just make the fucker work right the first time right out of the box. Stop loading it up with bull-shit programs and they'll be plenty fast enough. You know damn well what programs I'm talking about that are engineered to automatically load when the computer starts thus causing it to slow down. Regular people don't even know they're being screwed. Anymore I can't get Quick Time to stop auto-starting and why the fuck do I need Quick Time if I run on a PC. 1 program bitches! Make 1 program!

HOMEWORK BEFORE SHOPPING

Much to the contrary of what you think, nobody really wants to help you learn anything about consumer products anymore. Why am I writing about this? I have sold products in the retail sector for far too many years. The odds are that you have also sold retail at one point in your lives, so don't be stupid and inconsiderate. Ask your family, (who are always the authority on the subject anyway) what they think you should get. If you want to, I am giving you my permission to ask the salesman which one they think is the best for the money, but you have to trust them if you ask. Sometimes it's not unheard of for a sales rep to have received product knowledge training. Sometimes what they received was product embellishments. Who's to say? They also get to see what comes back and they get to know which brands are trash, so please don't disregard their opinions when they offer them.

CHANGE

The state of consumer products is in a constant flux. You must understand that big companies DO NOT CARE ABOUT YOU, and they do not care what features you want or don't want on your items. Sure they have a consumer opinion line, but it's not manned by a human and never gets checked. It's strictly for PR reasons and to make you feel better. If big corporations want to hire me as a consumer advocate or as a consultant for research and development then that would be great. Believe me; I have many bitches about more things than the average person. There are a few companies in particular that could use my help. Sony, Taco Bell, and Toyota to name a few are all doing just fine, but they are missing a few really obvious things that would put them over the top in both the sales and customer loyalty / satisfaction categories.

MOVING INTO THE FUTURE

Change IS good. If you don't like change and don't want to move into the future then you are a loser! You can't stop time or progress anymore than you can stop yourself from dying. If you could cheat death and had the money to start your own company that would only make the same things forever, then you would have earned yourself the right to live in the past. Can you do that?

Here is the rule plain and simple. You are not supposed to really believe this of course because it is bad for retail sales, but it is the truth. Everything electronic is basically made by one of a handful of major companies. That's why quality sucks. If one conglomerate owns 12 major brands then they can't survive if they don't cut back on jobs, quality assurance and materials costs. The same applies to automakers, power tools, cookware, furniture and types of candy. If you buy only the top of the line then at least you are assured of reputation, which is the one thing companies cling to in order to keep them positioned as a market leader and a winner of sales. If they give up the reputation for quality in their main product line then they are sunk.

TOO MANY CHOICES

Most companies do offer a lesser quality product because they want to capture business from both ends. I just don't like that we have so many things to look at. I want no more than 6 varieties of anything. Within those 6 I would like them to be broken down in pairs of 2 as *Cheap / Fair / Good*. Not Good / Better / Best, oh no because we all know that "Good" really isn't good at all. It's just a friendly way of saying cheap. If you can't afford the good stuff then don't just collect crap for the sake of feeling wealthy.

DON'T BE CHEAP

If you're poor you do have the God given right to complain about it. No one can take that away from you, nor should they. Rich people and those who win the lottery should not be so tight assed all the time. Go rent Brewster's Millions and act like that. Tip the people who work at Target very heavily. That's a cool store and they deserve some better pay. Employ someone as a limo driver and assistant at $30,000 a year. It won't kill you and it will change someone else's life. You're so damn stingy and really, can you take it with you? Besides, your children probably need to make their own way in life. Everyone hates rich kids. They act like fags. This is my point. On the other end of the spectrum, I really like Mexicans but they are always asking for a discount. Knock it off!

DESIGNING YOUR LIFE

This brings me to my next point. *Personal Growth Consultation* is the wave of the future. Remember and tell all of your friends that I coined this phrase. As you are reading this, I am officially declaring myself to be the first *Personal Growth Consultant* in history. Actually, should you or your business be in need of a consultant of any kind than you may contact my publicist or refer to my website. I will help you be cool and live the life you deserve if you really want to be a better person. Not being sarcastic here, seriously please contact me. We need more sharp razors in the toolbox.

Lifestyle Coordination is a very similar task that I should also endeavor to undertake as soon as publishing has been completed. The two titles are really the same thing in many respects except for that *Lifestyle Coordinator* will probably be for clients who are already vain. Mind you there is nothing wrong with a little vanity. Style; as it applies to your life is about knowing what is valuable and of personal importance and then striving to enhance your being by eliminating everything else. It is about listening to the person inside of you and not ignoring those suggestions. Take this for example. I don't believe that anybody in their true heart of hearts wants to drive a sedan. They're ugly and small. Even an older person wants something with room to breathe. Now there is a market for super small cars like the once great Honda CRX, but sedans just need to go. Free advice here...don't buy a sedan. You are only limiting your own potential on many levels. There are so many other, much cooler vehicles out there like the gas sucking Jeep or the Corvette.

Another example of a lifestyle that many people do not fully appreciate regards drinking. Drinking on the job should be allowed in the U.S. There exists a "right drink" for every person and every time. There is joy to be taken from living in a world when you know that and can act upon it. It is also a good idea to have the proper tools. I would encourage everyone to find their own personal favorite beverage holder and take it with you when you leave home. Open Container Law my ass. As much as you may not think so, people will have no choice but to admire your courage for making such a bold statement in a tight-assed world.

I hope you feel the necessity in your life to make a change. My services can help you overcome things like shyness with the opposite sex, poise / posture, attitude, direction, lack of class, marital problems, sexual dysfunction, obesity or anything else but you have to be willing to spend a few dollars and to make a change. Never be afraid of what another person might say. By my own admission I am far too relaxed for my own good and I admittedly have someone else dress me when I play for real. I have a fashion block in my mind and so I always trust the judgment of a woman. We can call in a specialist for you if you are a man too. Ladies, please do not be afraid or think that you are too good to have a *Lifestyle Coordinator* or *Personal Growth*

Consultant. Give me a call; even if you think you are rat face ugly, I can help.

HAIR REMOVAL

I have mentioned this subject in the sex chapter, but I must preach the glories of hair removal here as well. What are we, apes? We share certain characteristics. As for men, we can tend to share more than a few. One of these is the nasty collection of nappy curly hairs on our backs. Now I personally do not have this problem. I will admit to having a few random hairs by my shoulders every now and again but they are not shown the light of day. They are picked or shaved quickly.

I understand that it is a curse to have a hairy back or one with two thick stripes of hair (this is so nasty to even think about) but don't you feel obligated in some way to do something about it? I see men all the time riding their bikes or hiking or just even at the grocery store with either no shirts on or big ol' wads of hair coming out through the neck hole.

That is just not right.

Get a hot wax job done. Yeah it's gonna hurt so you might want to go to the store and get a bottle of Jack Daniels Whisky or whatever comforts you in your hours of need, but then it's gone and you can have a good time for at least a week or two before it starts to grow back.

What's even better is laser surgery-removal. I would like to have this done to my neckline and my fantastic pelvic region. The theory here is to kill off the follicles so that it never grows back. Hell yeah. Damn straight I would have that done, especially if I had a hairy, out-of-control back and arms.   Don't punish yourselves any further men. Go get it done. Now it can be a little expensive but it is going to change your life and I would imagine that if your doctor would describe your hairiness as a condition then your insurance might pick up at least part of the tab. You should also be aware that you may have to go back for as many as four treatments but then they are d-a-y-d dead as they say in the south. Problem solved and you have done your community a great service.

HOMELESSNESS

STAY THE FUCK OFF THE STREET CORNERS!!!!!!! This is really a basic violation of my rights. I want you gone from my sight! Permanently! No, I do not now, nor have I ever felt sorry for you. I feel sorry for me having to look at you. I applaud the states that have made it illegal to be a bum and approach you or ask for anything. Don't hold up signs to people in cars. They want to get out and punch you. It's one thing to not want to work. We can all understand and appreciate that working for somebody else mostly bites a big rubber cock made in China. I myself am inherently lazy. If you want to be a hobo, that's fine. Just accept the fact that you are going to have to eat trash and steal the fruit from trees. Just do not bother me.

I would rather die first than to beg. Begging is pointless and unnecessary in this day and age. There are places you can go to clean up and get help. Until then, keep your filthy broken ass out of the line of vision. People will help you! I will give you whatever help you need. I will not give you cash.

Let me tell a brief story: I was in the parking lot of a Home Depot in Aurora, CO one day doing my job. A man got out of his car and asked me for help. Three things were undeniable. He was old (he said 62), he was skinny (about 90lbs.) and he very much looked the part of having been beaten down. When he approached me the first words out of his mouth were "Pardon me Sir, God bless you. I need some help." We talked and he did in fact ask me for some money. I literally do not carry cash as a matter of principle for this reason alone. We were about 5 blocks from my church, where we had a mission outreach program just for this kind of thing and I knew the head Pastor. He asked me if I could go to the ATM. I told him we could leave right now and I would take him there and get him all the supplies and food he needed and it wouldn't have to be repaid. When this old man realized he wasn't getting a penny out of me in his hand, he got back in his car and drove off without a word. Didn't even end the conversation! Well having the short fuse that I do, I proceeded to yell "*You have a nice day and thank you for lying. I hope you go home in shame Sir. Pray not to burn in Hell for blaspheming!*"

It seems like such a simple issue. Why can't people have more self respect? I'm not exactly opposed to genocide / persecution and you people wonder why? It's because I have no faith in mankind. Lucky for you I'm not the Judge or the one pulling the trigger.

The other thing is the piss smell. Can't you people find a way to not smell like you shot it straight up at your chin? Other people can smell you from a hundred feet away and you shouldn't be allowed in stores. Find a river or something! If you must be a bum, I can tell you how to do it with some dignity and class. There are a few necessities that you should procure before you can successfully pull it off.

- 1 straight edge razor
- 1 multi-purpose stainless steel eating tool for camping
- 1 well-lined and presentable backpack or laptop case
- 1 nice large heavy beach towel
- 1 personal swimmers' shammy
- 1 pair of good looking sun glasses

- 3 changes of fresh clothes with no holes in them consisting of at least 1 collared shirt and 1 dress coat

You can do anything you want including sleep on the grass if you look like a professional who's just lounging. For the rest of the stuff (if you feel must collect it) you should get a Rubbermaid tub and bury it somewhere that doesn't get a lot of human traffic. Cover it with some leaves and shit. Leave a note that says, "This junk belongs to a bum. It's all I have so please respect me and don't mess with it."

I am slightly amused that the word "bum's" has an apostrophe denoting ownership of something to a bum. Irony is an awesome thing.

Nobody owes you anything. You can get a job even if you don't have legs. Now to get on with your bum life and stop begging, you will need a reliable source of food. After cleaning up, get a part time job at a fast food place. Work the lunch rush for three hours or something. That way you can get fed a good meal for almost nothing and you're not an eyesore for that time frame. Then go over to your local mall. Maybe get a small job there too. Work yourself in good with the security guards. Maybe find yourself a nice little mall nook that nobody knows about to make your home. Malls offer a lot of things including good protection from the elements. There are usually lots of bushes or things to hide behind.

Try to take your showers in the mornings. Volunteer to hose down the parking lot or driveway of some business and just make sure that you get a little wet in the process. They might even give you a leftover donut for breakfast.

Just a couple of other things: Cut your freakin' hair off, even if you're a girl. It's one less thing to worry about. People will not ask you if you have a disease. Stop pushing carts around with useless crap in it.   Recycling is not a fast enough method of money gathering for you people.

The rest of this is about housing the homeless population, which will disappear once I am in charge.   If the homeless who are willing to work are given training, jobs and guidance, they will in fact build homes for themselves. Hey, all of a sudden they have a decent sum of cash and a roof.   It is starting in some states. Sweat equity it is called, but it is a slow moving vehicle. The work crews don't have enough bums in them. Once a crew finishes one bum's house then they could move on to the next bum's house. Give the construction company huge breaks and incentives to cooperate.

There are mountains of school closings around the nation. So let's give them the closed schools (under strict supervision) to live in. Come on Habitat for Humanity! What's great about this idea is that there are many rooms, usually a playground and a fence to keep them out of sight, and a gymnasium with SHOWERS! FREE SHOWERS FOR ALL! Then once the doorman has checked to make sure they are not overly stinky, they can come out into the world. It's not a prison, it's a free home with a bed or cot or something, where no one will ask you to do anything but sit around and t
alk about the good old days. I'm not too concerned about them using the kitchen. They can cook if they want to. That fast food job option becomes a reality real fast once you're clean and have a residence.

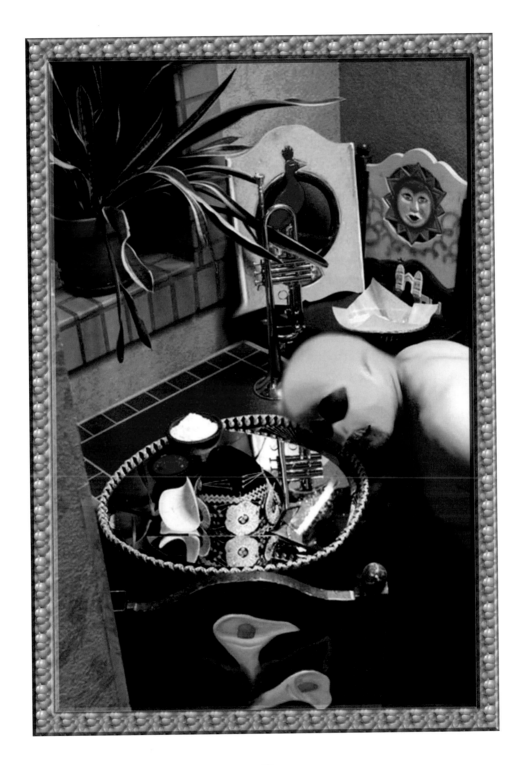

"ILLEGAL ALIENS"

This picture was supposed to be called Higher Love the portrait of an Alien woman and Human man who had just completed making inter-species love and are now joined in a vertical embrace. I mention this to you for future Copyright protection. I was going to have a ridiculous physical male specimen to represent the fact that even the best, the most perfect among us is not immune to the effects of love and that it is possible to transcend species if the mind is willing. Love can be blind even if you have rather large eyes. The other notable suggestion would have been that the man is pregnant rather than the alien woman because she is too skinny. The theory behind many supposed abductions is that various races are attempting to combine our species so that we can co-habituate the same planet with less risk for disease. I'll get that pic taken too. You just wait.

Since I wasn't able to get the shot I wanted because the tiny model wouldn't cooperate and show her nipples (God only knows why) my good friend "Doty" stepped up to the plate with this gem. If you're either a Mexican or a U.S. Citizen & this doesn't offend you, then you're clearly numb to the world. A space alien who got fat off of buttery burritos doing cocaine on a sombrero! Come on? That's funny all day long! Aliens like to party too. You can't be ignorant and think that all they do is work on science projects. Read the damn chapter. They party and they fuck. Let's get it on!!!!!

Photography: Parrish Douglas

Concept By: David Doty

ALIENS and U.F.O.'s

CHAPTER III

Acclimation time...yes! I am certainly not an authority on the subject, although bizarre things happen to me all the time. I think they enjoy stealing a variety of my stuff such as keys. I am convinced they freeze time in my area to do this and then they wait until I get really mad before they put the object in question back in plain view where I will find it. Oh I get so mad, and you swear up and down that you know exactly where you put things. I also think they have put at least 2 RFID style tracking chips in my body so they can find me and fuck with me at a moment's notice when they're bored.

I don't have to be an expert and I don't have to quote any sources. There are so many people out there writing on this subject that I don't even need to prove credibility! You can't hide from it. I am merely collaborating efforts on your behalf. This chapter was originally written solely for the purpose of inspiring thought. In all fairness, you might have trouble swallowing some of this stuff. The information here is a reiteration of things I have read or learned in college. I did have an astrology professor who claimed to do high level contract work for the government on this subject. As a means of release, he loved sharing information that he wasn't supposed to. Many of the persons who have shared their knowledge are understandably afraid to speak in public and still others have embraced it. No one should be condemned or put down for their beliefs though, whether it is on this subject or any other. It is only through the avenues of free speech that we can continue to evolve our minds.

Aren't you just about ready to know the truth about aliens? Indelibly there is an answer and a truth. Elect me President and I will tell you everything. At the very least I should be appointed Minister for Extra-Terrestrial Affairs under this administration. What are we still going to live in the dark ages for another 60 years or more, ignoring everything we hear? I will be dead by then and I would like to know by physical evidence before that time comes. There is a reason that so many movies and television shows are produced about alien races. That reason is to knock down public fear in order to prepare you for integration. C'mon, that's *EXACTLY* why they make a crap-load of movies about it.

Let's get it on I say! I want to live in the future where we share technology and have flying cars and light sabers. That would kick ass! Claims have been made that multiple governments coerce the film making efforts in their countries. The first documented Hollywood / Government collaboration is said to have been the 1951 original version of "The Day the Earth Stood Still". This practice continues to this day and is now so vivid that we don't have to imagine anymore. Not surprisingly, that film was just remade while I was in editing of this project. By the way, none of your favorite television series are exempt either. Now we even have entire channels on TV dedicated to this subject and more channels such as History run regular documentaries. I even watched one show dedicated to the discovery of Atlantis in which one American scientist claims that entire culture was completely alien and they already did mix their genetic structures with ours as far back as 11,000 years ago. I understand that society is being prepped for integration by this gradual dissemination of information. For fuck's sake already, somebody just be responsible and make the official announcement! I did hear that France and possibly Russia are at least leading the way by de-classifying 100% of their documents. They're not saying anything more about them, but they have been released for viewing since 2006.

So as far as living with aliens goes, I would even date an alien chick if I weren't involved at the time when we initiate public contact. As long as disease testing is kept under control and studied, I'd probably have sex with one too. I'm sure they have inner beauty just like many of our wives and husbands. Look at your mate. Really, how outwardly attractive are they? How often do you have sex with that? Yikes!

GET READY...HERE THEY COME

Why don't they ever appear in broad daylight? Why don't they fly at lower altitudes and slowly so that someone could distinguish what they are? If they want to study us, why do they not make a scheduled announcement asking for volunteers? They should place an ad on the Internet requesting to the world which types of people they would like to focus on. I'm sure that volunteers by the hundreds would line up for a knowledge exchange. Even at a basic level. If they or our governments are afraid of a sweeping alien hysteria then why not hold a telecast / public meeting in broad daylight, with plenty of security and bullet proof "Pope Glass" in a huge public place with lots of witnesses just to say... *"Hi, were here. We don't want to scare anybody. Don't hurt us and we won't hurt you. OK, thanks for your time but we've got to go now. We'll give spaceship rides in the future. Stay cool."*

CLOSE ENCOUNTER

I have had a personal experience that scared me shitless, literally. It took place about 8 years after I wrote 228 pages of this book so this section is obviously an amendment to the original chapter layout. Based on things I wrote down afterward, this happened on the night of June 12th 2006. I'll relate it as best I can.

I was camping for 3 days with about 10 or 12 other guys in the mountains west of Salida, CO. The first 2 nights went off without a hitch. On the 3rd night it was warmer and I chose to sleep in a hammock that was away from the campsite about 100 feet into the woods, so not that far. I am a light sleeper. I woke up at 2am and looked at my watch as a habit so this probably occurred at about 3:30am knowing that it takes me a while to go back to sleep. The next time I woke up it was to the sound of something loud like a semi-truck crashing through the trees. Somebody may have run over something with their camper, I don't know. I didn't really care at the time and that's not what scared me.

A few minutes later a hand held red light passed over my closed eyelids several times. From that moment and for the next 4 hours I could hear and see directly in front of me, but I could not otherwise move my eyes and I was completely paralyzed. I remember hearing several voices quietly talking to each other in a language that was not English. One of them did speak to me enough that I recognized that they did not intend to harm me. In my peripheral vision I could see their heads, but not clearly. My right arm was lifted out from a blanket that was on top of my sleeping bag. Then I saw the arm and hand of a creature with 3 fingers touch the end of my fingers. They held it for a little while and the sense I got was very peaceful. Then they put my arm down and communicated that was all. I couldn't move. It wasn't until after everyone else had woken up and was stirring about that I was able to get up. The effect wore off slowly and I had extreme difficulty walking and going to the bathroom that morning. I did ask around (since I'm not shy) but no one else claimed to have heard anything. I also could not find any evidence of a crash.

So that's my 3rd Kind Encounter story. I swear to you that is the way I remember it, verbatim. Take it or leave it. I get the feeling that I personally have been abducted about 5 or 6 times. They seem to enjoy tracking me, I don't know.

I believe that there are more different types of aliens running around than we have bones in our body. I believe that we have been visited or at least watched since near the creation of human life on our world whenever it was (totally irrelevant). Really, why is that not possible?

I do not believe that there are any evil races of beings, only evil individuals. Even if giant intelligent bugs invade the earth, just because they're hungry doesn't mean they're evil. I'm sure if you asked a cow, chicken or baby sheep they'd think we are evil. This raises an interesting point that perhaps I'll explore sometime in the future. Why doesn't anyone make a movie about malevolent farm-type animals invading the earth? Most of us can remember the series "V" (if you can't PLEASE rent it). I guess lizards are as close as it will ever come. More on "V" in a minute!

GRAYS

I'm going to speak for now about "the Grays". Again, I'm not a "Ufologist" but it is interesting and I like to read and learn things. So there is a lot to be told of the plight of the Grays. Apparently they have all but destroyed their home world with pollution, misuse of natural resources and abuse of technology. They are supposedly now involved with the human race in an effort to create a hybrid species for their future generations in an effort to regain a part of what they have lost in terms of emotionality. Apparently they are rather cold beings who do a lot of work and don't have a lot of fun. It is also an effort to become closer to

God, something that they believe in, but they feel they have reached an impasse in their spiritual evolution.

As for the eyes, since the time when the outward appearance of their planet was destroyed they have moved underground. The lack of natural sunlight has caused them to develop their optical sensory organs to the point of needing little light. This might help to explain why they operate very little during the day hours here on earth. Popular belief is now such that the large eyes are actually very good sunglasses that they developed for use here. They may not wear much else for suits or clothing. I don't personally believe that the grays run around our planet naked because they are skinny and would therefore be cold. Maybe the away teams have Viking attitudes though.

Their heads are by all accounts too large for their bodies. It is generally accepted that they are able to communicate telepathically, however I do not see the connection between telepathy and a large cranium. Since as humans we only use an average of 10% of our brains ability, it seems logical that we would have the ability to develop and use telepathy of our own without the need to increase our cranial chamber. Over time perhaps the brain as an independent organ would feel the need to grow and generations later a change would be seen. That would not be improbable.

It has come to my attention that although their physical bodies are not massive or sexually intriguing, that they do have one discernible advantage and one big disadvantage.

On the up side, apparently they no longer have the need or even the capacity to defecate. This could be completely rumor. Don't get too excited, I'm just relating. I find this personally amazing and cool if it were to be true. This is something I really would like to see happen to humans. It's such a nasty thing to have to participate in. Even at its best when you have a bidet, it still seems pointless to me. Why do I bother to eat if I'm only going to lose half of it in a few hours? When I eat something I want my body to use it all. Make me more muscles or do something creative with it like grow a few more penises so that there is always one ready to go. Most guys can go again a few minutes after they ejaculate, but by then the mood is already ruined. And who can't use bigger muscles huh?

On the down side (in a super segue) from what I understand, the Grays have lots of sexual issues! First of all, I have heard that their sexual organs are all but shriveled and are only used for bird-like waste disposal. There still is a definition between male and female, although it doesn't matter because reproduction is all controlled by test-tube. For those of you who haven't done much reading about the subject prior to this, here is the supposed reason they have switched, by choice, to this type of creation methodology.

At one time the Grey's were just sex machines. They did each other left and right in the streets. They did their own cousins and sisters. They did it on their work breaks with their fellow employees in front of the others and sometimes in groups. They did it so much that they finally came to a point where disease ran rampant and they were killing themselves off at an alarming rate. Coupled with other social decline, a high-level decision was made to begin tube style reproduction. Using this method they could engineer their next generations to all be very similar in intelligence and abilities, but lacking so much sexual desire. Thus they would create a superior work force and social harmony through a lack of interest. By that I mean that they even engineered their genitals to be less productive and functional over time.

Now you can believe what you like. Personally I don't think it is too far from the truth. I mean why not? Why couldn't it have happened that way? I think that maybe in one of my past lives that I was one of the sexually dominant on their planet. (Dominant meaning about 3 inches)

ACTUAL MARTIANS!

Once again, this chapter is at least 90% hearsay, but you have to believe something. There is a lot of evidence that suggests that there once was humanoid life on Mars. You can find many books in your local bookstore in or near the metaphysical, astrological, or science sections that can tell you more. The latest I have read is that they are still alive as a race, not thriving at all, but surviving in part thanks to other alien races and shared technology that I will cover next. This information comes by way of research in what some people might call Astral Projection.

What do they look like? Well according to several publications, the chances of you already having seen one are better than you winning the lottery. Supposedly they are taller on the average than we are, contrary to prior opinion. The best way to describe them would be crack-babies. They are very slender as a race, with eyes only slightly further apart. I could only assume their skin pigmentation would make them look like a pale-blue Caucasian. If this were the case, it would be due to a lack of natural sunlight. Supposedly they have been living underground, under various mountain ranges in the central U.S. and abroad. There could still be a group under the Martian surface, I am not sure.

What happened to them? Well, the asteroid theory for one. It did not strike the planet's surface. Instead it came dangerously close, creating a rift in the atmosphere, which eventually collapsed. It did leave them with enough time however to save a few groups of people. Later, either the Grays or a similar race took pity and helped to move the species, giving them accelerated technology as well to help them adapt, survive and remain hidden. That's all I know about that.

OTHER RACES

This is dissemination of knowledge from direct and ongoing contact with the U.S. Government, and yes it includes some area 51 stuff.

In real life there are more groups of aliens than we care to admit (officially 1 is more than we care to admit). Most note worthy are the group referenced in "Close Encounters of the Third Kind". There is a section at the very end of the movie where 12 astronauts + 1 civilian are taken in the ship to another planet. A version of this really happened, minus the 1 civilian going and the aliens left one of their own here on Earth.   This group is called the Ebens. (Almost all of the names I have heard are acronyms for something. I'll let you look those up for yourself.)

The Ebens are the oldest group that we know of and they are the most advanced so far as we are aware. It is said that they have had their hands in creating entire other races by genetic experiment. This is to say that they are cloners.

According to the website I read the Eben have created at least 4 other unique species. Three of them have "Grey" characteristics with some distinctions. They also created a race that resembles lizards and not so friendly. I believe there are 6 to 8 more in addition to that. Some races were from earlier time periods.

I made mention earlier to the TV mini-series "V" which stood for "visitors". In this drama, gigantic ships came to earth bearing beings that were humanoid and in fact appeared to be human for a good long time. They claimed that their home plant had run out of water and that they wanted to use some of ours. As it turned out they were actually harvesting humans for food storage purposes. (The scene where you see the storage chamber was particularly cool for its time) Anyway, war erupts and so on and so forth.

Why couldn't there be a reptilian group as well? They have been crawling around for a lot longer than we have. They are probably here now as well and working with humans (possibly against their will, possibly not) to achieve some future goal.

I also now hear tell that some aliens are inter-dimensional demons. Yes this does come from the Internet. I say; no comment. Maybe but I could care less. I only care about the ones I can play rugby with and win against.

This is not meant to alarm anyone, just merely to assist your awareness that there are several distinctly different groups of aliens that may be operating on earth. Have a nice day. :)

NEW MEXICO

There are about a dozen other recognized crash sites you know. Anyway, all of the cool sightings happen around high plains and deserts for a reason. It's because people in cities don't bathe enough and they can smell us from space. My good friend and stunt double, M. Roderick Kramer III Esq. has never been abducted and he definitely smells like goat piss. We love him though. Well supposedly desert climates closely resemble the preferred living terrain on many of these other planets. Of course they have polar ice caps and nasty hot regions and jungles. If we put in a huge theme park and a nice lake between Albuquerque and Santa Fe I think New Mexico would really take off as an inter-species real estate hub.

It is rumored on the SERPO.org website that the next scheduled visit where we all sit down and have Oreo™ cookies and milk will be on Thursday, November 11th at some Nevada test location. This is all open to change of course. They supposedly snuck in a meeting in 2009 on the U.S. military island of Johnston Atoll in the Pacific. It still takes some time to travel here and this group is not operating from a moon base as one of the 3 Gray groups supposedly are. In attendance will not only be members of several world governments but the Pope as well.

YOU BETTER INVITE ME YOU GOVERNMENT FUCKS!!!

I am excited to be a part of the dissemination of information to the public that will inevitably lead to a greater consciousness.

ALIEN TECHNOLOGY

One of the principle reasons that I believe aliens are visiting our planet is that we have reached the point where we can put nipples on our department store mannequins. Many of them even look better than real humans. You know you want to touch them. Everyone does. Even women. I think that we owe it to ourselves to use this development in some kind of information trade on their vehicles.

Laser guns and plasma based energy swords I highly doubt are strapped to the side of every alien. I do think that something similar to a laser gun or pulse weapon exists, but that it's our current government that's working on those weapons. There are sources that have stated after their retirement that the Lockheed-Martin "Skunk Works" already possesses almost every piece of technology that we have seen in the movies.

Telepathy and telekinesis or psycho kinesis (PK) as it is often called are very real and very possible. I do not have this gift available to me as of yet, but if you know someone who has reached that plateau please have him or her set up shop, call me and start teaching. We didn't dream up telepathy or telekinesis as something for a science-fiction movie. If we are only using 10% of our brains capability on the average, don't you think it might be a good idea to develop and use the rest? I want that gift very badly. More than you can imagine. I would do almost anything for it.

Now for their other technological developments such as ships: It was told to me by a fairly believable authority on space, science and the physical universal laws, that the craft used by the Grays have certain spatial altering abilities. One of these allows their craft and the contents within to be "phase shifted" in such a manner as to allow them to pass through things like the side of a mountain or buildings for example. This would be what the Martians are supposedly utilizing to remain hidden underground, quite likely on their home world as well.

The ships power supply and flight drive run on something akin to a gravity well (if I remember correctly). It could be gyroscopic and magnetic in nature as well, it really was about 20 years ago that I learned this. Anyhow, what allows them to travel such distances without growing old is this "well device", not a "warp drive" per say.

Here's how it works; visualize a piece of paper as representing a flat cross-section of the galaxy. Instead of trying to traverse this entire distance, what they are able to do is to fold space over, much like making the piece of paper into a cylinder by placing the ends together. Then, your starting point and your destination are much closer together and they just make the shorter hop as it was across to the other side. Once there, space along that line unfolds. This makes possible for them a trip that would have taken several hundred years in only a few minutes or hours. It makes sense doesn't it? I have no idea how to build the thing. I'm just the messenger, but I do think it's a pretty sweet idea.

There are rumored to be many types of craft with many different propulsion systems; hence the different variety of lighting schemes that have been reported. I could not tell you how most of the others work but I do recall seeing several things on the History Channel. Those guys are specialists on taking one topic and stretching it out for 3 seasons. I know what a "teaser" is in terms of a commercial break and you need to knock that crap off. I only have about 20 minutes a day for television anyway and I require mindless violence and cartoons to fill at least half of that.

COMMUNICATIONS DEVICES

When you think about all the different telephone and cellular companies out there, do you get a little discouraged? I do, especially since they do their best to make gaining your business an unholy war. They bombard you in your home with calls at the most inappropriate times and you have to hear it on the radio and TV in every other commercial. It's nonsense. When are we just going to switch to one global communications network and act like adults?

Did I mention that the service should be free? Well I'm sure you'll agree that it should, with restrictions of course for the people that can't ever shut up. I'll even agree to purchase the little device, because after all I would be the one to give it wear and tear. It just sucks that in our current state of world greed we can't just buy one phone and start using it everywhere in the world. Why does it cost $2.13 per minute to call someone in Taiwan? We also have to "select a plan" and commit ourselves to bad service for entirely too long.

I am thinking of course of something similar to what used in the ever-popular Star Trek series. Something on that scale would probably have to be overseen by the new world government for it to work. Let us understand also that the communications array in Star Trek dealt with a mere 2000 crew members (give or take) (mostly take), and that on earth we have some 7 billion people. It could be done though. We just need a centralized organization, a few dedicated satellites and a little time, that's all. **Opinion** I would like to publicly say for the record that I believe Qwest to have the worst customer service of any company in the nation today. Qwest can send a representative to my house to suck my ass! That is all...

FOOD

Apparently almost all of the Grays are now vegetarians, and nutritional pill takers to boot. I could be wrong here but I've heard that they have genetically engineered themselves and their food supplies so that "pooping" is no longer necessary. I say good for them. Through the power of meditation and my mind I have altered my body to indeed use most of what I eat so that at the most I only have to go once a day. I have been known to go for as many as 3 days while still eating quite a bit so here again evolution to something like that is possible. Massive amounts of fiber helps.

The Grays, do not have an anus, (or so I have been told). Since their bodies utilize a much greater percentage of what they digest they do not need one. They dispose of their waste in a quasi-liquid form much like a bird does, through their urinary tract. Again I could be wrong, but if a Government official would like to correct me on that point it would certainly be welcome because that would be an admission of guilt.

The point is that intelligent races believe it's wrong to kill a living animal in order to eat it. Besides it's very gross. I would like to see every American who likes their beef, go out and personally slaughter and prepare a dead cow carcass. Do you think you could do it? If the answer is no, then you need to rethink your position. How righteous is your cause if you yourself are a hypocrite?

If the answer is yes, then more power to you. Go on and have a good time. I won't bother you anymore. You would have earned it.

If I were a Native-American living on the plains before we had technology, I'd be a berry picker. I'd pick berries all the daylong. When I wasn't doing that, I'd be fighting with the other tribesman. I'd fight and I'd be a mean son-of-a-bitch just so I wouldn't have to hear about not eating meat all the time. My grass diet would keep me plenty strong. I might even be a lone wolf if my tribe banished me. But then I'd have to go to the neighboring village and give away all of their secrets or perhaps lead a silent raid to exact my revenge.

At any rate, the Gray's couldn't eat meat anymore even if they wanted to. They no longer develop their molar teeth that would allow them to grind the meat once it is bitten off. Also the amount of hard to digest proteins in their little bodies would send them to the hospital immediately, doubled over in pain. Not having eaten meat for a while their stomachs could not process it without causing large turds which they physically could not pass.

ALIEN RELIGIOUS BELIEFS

Why couldn't an alien race believe in the same things we do? It's funny how we attach human characteristics to them so that we can make them more identifiable. Clearly they are advanced well beyond us so it stands to reason that they should know one or maybe two things more about God than we do. The apparent age of their race alone would dictate that.

Here's what I've read. There's not much to argue about here. I guess they have the same Jesus figure and same mostly everything. It is fair to say that the son of God would have visited their planet first and then either made a repeat visit to earth and the other planets. It is suggested in some circles that the Ebens assisted in portraying Jesus on earth for the purpose of spreading their religion. It's a little over the top but not unlike sending missionaries to remote jungles where the inhabitants have no clue what's going on. That and the fact that every old culture in the world has made portraits of creatures that descend from the sky _in vehicles_. Even the theory of Immaculate Conception is not out of the realm of possibility for them. If they can abduct and impregnate us now, then certainly it could have happened before.

INTERNET SEARCH HOMEWORK

Here are some key words. This will give you more than enough entertainment for at least a week. Go have fun.

1) Zeta-Reticuli
2) Remote Viewing
3) Levitation
4) Alien Abductions
5) Lockheed Martin Skunk Works
6) Telepathy
7) Psycho kinesis

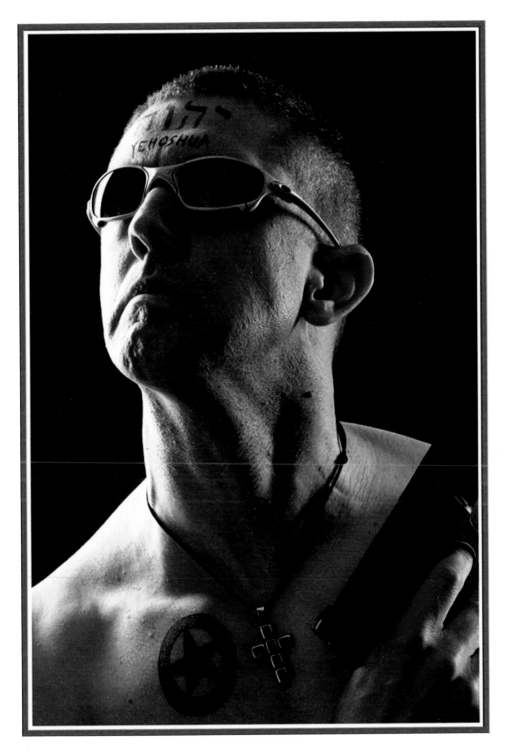

Leaders of Tomorrow

For those of you who aren't Jewish and don't get the deep symbolism contained within; this picture is about the end of days and the people who may be a part of the army of God. Let me break it down for you: These are the people who might be fighting for our souls. The Hebrew letters in blood red roughly translate into God: the "I am" indicating ownership. Below in the tradition of Revelation is the name Jesus in Hebrew (but with English letters) *as best as I can* translate from the Old Testament. Notice the cross which is a direct affront to the Jewish belief that Jesus is not the savior, and the gun that signifies man's attempt to control by "very limited" power. Tatted Marshal badge: that also represents the earthly belief in the authority of man. My facial expression represents the inner struggles of man. We have an evil nature and must fight to do good. Everything is in contrast. That's what makes this a great shot! I paid $300 bones for the Oakley glasses so they're just in there for the cool factor.

As it pertains to the future; really I feel our collective ugly, stinking; good for very little children whom we cannot trust to take out the trash are incapable of accomplishing very much in the way of humanitarianism or Godliness. Call me a cynic but I don't have faith in us, let alone them. So what exactly are we going to do about the future? Pro'lly get blown to purgatory; even if we are believers. Be ready and have fun with that!

Date Taken: September, 2009

Location: Denver, CO / DeSciose Studios Complex

Concept By: Parrish Douglas – stud form

Photo and Edit by: Nicholas DeSciose/Photographer-Filmmaker

GOVERNMENT & LAW

CHAPTER IV

I want to be the first President-elect for the planet earth. This planet needs one central body that acts for the good of mankind and we are but children in the cosmos until this happens. I don't care about the damn money or power; I just want to do what's right for us on this planet as a global society.

> ➢ STOP.   Don't get all bent out of shape.

If you haven't already figured it out; R E A D   S L O W L Y. You will now observe that I go between the political lines like a drunk driver with a near death 2.0 blood/alcohol content. It will be easier and more pleasant for you to read the next 4 chapters if you can set aside your political party associations and any other ties you may have to our conventional systems. Now go get a beer and come back...

Welcome back. What is it about the government of the United States of America that we love? What are the things we hate? Why are there so many things we hate? Why do we tolerate corruption? Why can't the government talk less and do more? Why do we still have so many problems with taxation?

I am a citizen of the Earth, not of the United States. I would denounce myself anytime if it meant that I could travel more freely and not be taxed for shit I don't care about. I did have to buy all of my guns here before publishing though because they ask you if you have ever denounced your citizenship so they can put you on a potential terrorist black list. I'll have guns in multiple countries by the time this comes out and then I'm aiming to have triple citizenships.

I'm inserting a little about Communism here because I think that it is entirely misunderstood. To do it right you have to build a system from the ground up. One that doesn't punish the rich with over-taxation, but one that also legitimately works to help the poor. Slow down your reading <u>again</u> and follow me. The principals are sound. It's only the people who ran the system that ever gave it a bad name. Let's see here; general medical costs are paid, basic food supplies, housing for the poor and assignable jobs. The root of Communism really is designed to help the people. Americans like to raise a stink about things that are far away and people that appear to be different. That's flat out wrong America. We might have to revisit this one final time.

TALK SHOW BITCHES

This seems like an appropriate place to discuss something of great importance to me since it affects the next 4 chapters.

Why would I possibly call talk show hosts "bitches"? Maybe because they preach all the time? It never stops. They never have a kind word to say. They don't actually disseminate much information at all. It's hypocritical gum flapping. Their speeches are solely another form of entertainment. The worst episode of South Park™ is better than the best of their shows. I can't understand what they are yapping about because there isn't any silence to let it soak in. You are the cause of public outrage. When citizens get irate then their representatives get bent out of shape. The effect of your constant negativity spirals. That's why we have a lot of dissention about our government and we get very little change. People are opposed to working together before they even show up on Capitol Hill. I blame you.

Larry King I believe is a good man and people respect the fact that he has a wide variety on his show. I could hang with him. I also have immense respect for Dr. Laura Schlesinger. No, I speak negatively of Nancy Grace, "Pencil-Dick" Rush Limbaugh and Sean Hannity whom I think has the face of a backstabbing child molester. Actually I think he was spawned from one of Rush's hemorrhoids. There are others just as bad on local radio levels. How come Hannity's latest book (which should be titled "Tears of My Vagina") gets a 1.5 million copy first run press and mine does not? You don't get nipples in his book, only smelly vagina tears. WTF?

Grace; you shut your mouth or I will personally select a dirty sewer bum with scabies and Gono-Syphi-Herp-AIDS to fuck you in the ass. Maybe the bum can tag out with Bill O'Reilly just for humiliation and some extra kicks. I don't like you. I want your job so I can attempt to undo all the evil you have caused. You and Pelosi are born from the same ugly devil womb. I would rather listen to Delilah for 30 days straight than to have to see your cock-whore mouth on my television for 30 seconds. It's that bad.

The funny thing is I really don't have a reason to hate you (ALL) on a personal level. If you would just shut the fuck up and listen to somebody else speak we could be OK (as in Old Kinderhook 8th President). What's up now bitches? You know about that party?

TEA PARTY members; listen up. You need to contact me right now! You are on the verge of being considered serious but you need to stop making colossal blunders and get some advice from a visionary. I know you already dumped a bunch of money into

Sarah Palin but she is not qualified to represent you in the White House. She runs away from responsibility. Just consult me.

Back to business... what the fuck good have any of the talk show hosts ever done for the world? Really, I am talking about legitimate out of your comfort zone results. How many addicts have you driven to rehab after a 2am Taco Bell run? How many bills have you sponsored and introduced to congress? How many times have you even wiped your own piss from the urinal wall? You are useless and you take too much oxygen from the rest of us. Ever try broadcasting your show from a soup kitchen or a foster children's home on Christmas? You don't like my brand of sensitivity and civic duty? Go fuck yourself with a serving ladle.

I hereby challenge any damn one of you to put me on your show for the entire day length of the program, and...AND you also have to shut the hell up like a good moderator and not interrupt the guest. You can't negate the points I argue. I am that damn good. You can't take me down. You are in-valid as a group and furthermore I need for you to prove your worth as human beings by taking me to lunch at a strip club after the show. That is how you show respect for your guests.

THE PRESIDENCY

Since he was recently elected, I have to say at least 2 sentences about President Obama. God help him with the pile of crap he is taking on. He is almost guaranteed to win re-election because there is absolutely no way to fix all of our problems in 4 years (which he has already stated) and that is assuming that some more crap doesn't get thrown on top, which it will. Let's just hope we can stay out of war for that time. Good luck Mr. President and feel free to appoint me as one of your chief advisors. I will graciously accept.

That having been said, most of us or at least good percentages have always wanted to be the President. There are things about the country that we would all like to change. Maybe you would like to take action for a cause that you feel strongly about. If you have never heard it, go listen to the song "Vote for Me". It is by the group Chicago and is on their 11th Long-Play record album! I am laying claim to that right now as my 2016 campaign theme song.

I would love to be the leader of the free world. To have knowledge of every secret program ever run. I could then officially *and* with good conscience lie to rest the rumors of every conspiracy theory. That would of course cause an initial uproar because it would implicate every prior administration of covering things up in the supposed interest of the general public. The public wants to know and I would tell them everything!

There would be fear in the Oval Office but if you bring in your own trusted people you couldn't be touched. To have a group of personal secret service agents that will mop the floor with anyone who threatens me with a glare would be awesome. I don't need Air Force One, but a tank to drive myself through rush hour and a personal jet fighter. I would be the coolest President ever.

I believe that the American public has developed a fascination with their Presidents. We love to read about them, see them on TV, even create scenarios and pretend they actually happened. Sometimes they did. Why is it that we have not had a single (un-married) President in the history of our country? If we enjoy so much watching and following the escapades of such an individual, then why not elect a single man with whom the nation could be enamored and cheer for when he goes out with a woman. Elect someone who gives a kiss to the waitress who's serving him, or one who's not afraid to appear on the late night TV shows and talk about their personal lives. That's what all the stars do.

Maybe the President could even have girlfriends in each state or be given dates with the Miss USA pageant rep for each state.

For that matter why not have a single female President? I believe we are very close to having a female in the big chair at the White House. (Not Hillary Clinton or some actress!!! Give an unknown a chance.) Un-married heads of state are not an uncommon thing in other countries; it is just ours that puts so much emphasis on the structure.

This is a side tangent but it does at least pertain to the chapter. I would never have voted for either George W. Bush or Hilary Clinton and here's why. That allows for much power in one family. That yields corruption and there's not a shadow of doubt in my mind that both of these individuals and their families have been involved in some very underhanded things. I hear tell that Clinton is a relative to the Rockefellers. So that is the end of that! Internet search ROCKEFELLER SCANDAL and just see what comes up! I found 4 separate and distinct results.

As I said, I would like to be in office. I would like to work with a Congress and a House that was above reproach; a group of legislators that worked for not only the betterment of the country and its peoples, but for the rapid development of the entire world. I believe that we are a part of a cosmic society (albeit an inactive member). Once we can pull ourselves away from such ways of thinking as gas powered vehicles and eliminate issues of race, housing projects, and unacceptable pay, then we can concentrate on moving ahead as a planet.

When I run I don't plan on having any party affiliations. I think we have missed out on some excellent potential leaders because of narrow mindedness and party lines. I will tell you that I have voted Independent in the last 4 elections and I don't think that it is wasting a vote. Come on, you just have to not be a puss about your own opinions. Your vote does matter. At least Anderson (unofficially) won the 2 non-contiguous states in the 1980 election against Carter & Reagan. That was very forward thinking, but we let the momentum die. Officially he only won 6 + % of the popular vote. Don't question me! I remember watching the TV. I live for the color maps at election time! They divided HI & AK because Anderson didn't have enough to count and both the real parties wanted to save face.

If an Independent candidate ever hopes to win the office they have to start early. They have to hold regular campaign rallies for 2 years prior to the election and they have to be a master at communication and manipulating the media for their benefit.

Please! You've got to help me here! By buying this book and recommending it to everyone you know, you are at least spreading the word about the righteous cause of independent thinking. Do it for your planet and for your children's' future. Thank you.

NATIONAL DEBT

It occurred to me in editing that I had not explained the way our currency system works and why exactly we have such a huge national debt that we can't seem to settle. There's a reason for that. The banks don't want it settled. We've been keeping them afloat since the inception of the Federal Reserve. We have a treasury department and we do own and operate the U.S. Mints, however our government does not own the Federal Reserve. The FED in an independently owned bank that survives off the interest it makes from giving our government loans. This is a fucking nightmare to understand and I hate math so just take my word for it, you are being "schtionked" in the poop hole.

It only costs us 22 cents or so to print every dollar, so we actually make money on that branch of the government. The only items we lose money on printing is the penny and the nickel, so let's just eliminate those and make them collector items. The mint wants you to collect coins because it takes money out of circulation that they are told they have to replace. That's where we gain revenue. Pure and simple though …(I am talking boiled down to the bare oil)… as a nation we spend more than we can support with our own gold, so therefore we have to borrow money from a private bank called the FED and we owe them a metric shit-pile of interest. *What we need to do is take over the FED by eminent domain and subsequently erase ¾ of our own national debt.* End of story. Fuck yourself if you disagree!!!

We are in trouble because we have money printed that is backed by only so much gold. We don't actually trade in gold anymore, just fictitious shares of gold (not real weighable ounces). There is an important distinction. Gold is a finite, limited quantity unless you are a miner. It makes sense that there should only be so much money in circulation at one time but that should not be a variable. Unfortunately for us with the paper dollar system, we have variables.

National debt vs. budget deficit or surplus: A budget surplus has happened before and it could happen again. Let's say we ever stop fighting wars. Congress would still ask for a bunch of money; but if spending checks and balances are still in place then they won't need it all. The amount we need can be increased or reduced dramatically every year. It doesn't necessarily have to feed off itself from an interest aspect. Congress can simply ask for less while we also increase our Gross National Product. For example; we could sell our deformed children to the wealthy Chinese and create a whole new taxable export class.

The buying and selling of United States debt on the open market through U.S. Bonds either frees up or retracts the amount of cash flow coming through the Federal Reserve. *(Like I said...I fucking mental nightmare)!*

The U.S. Mint System has ABSOLUTELY, 100% the right to print up as much cash as they want to and dump it into the market. Problem is the value of the dollar then decreases. It's the biggest, gayest, most elaborate scheme on the planet and it all boils down to one thing; controlling the flow of money so that a very _few people become stinkingly rich_ and it's all legal. It's legal in every county, just some countries are better at managing the game than others.

What's the answer for you; the end user of cash? Don't live beyond your means and you won't get into trouble every time our money situation changes. Beyond that; stockpile tomato soup and good luck.

FORMING A ONE-NATION PLANET

I wrote the following paragraph in 1997 with no knowledge that such a task was in the planning stages. Truly, truly I say to you that I am a damn genius. Read this and I will explain what is currently transpiring in a few pages.

Obviously, a weak nation is not going to take over the rest of the planet by force. In terms of whether or not any strong country should take over everything, I don't think so. Rather the U.N. should come to a consensus on what a new form of world currency should be. All the nations in the U.N. should then all be required to accept this monetary change as well as that from their individual countries for a while. Of course, intelligent humans will voluntarily switch to the new currency and lead the way. That of the individual countries will soon after disappear. Exchange rates will be a thing of the past and really the only persons who would stand to be hurt by that are the people who take their high value monies and choose to live in third world countries. Everyone else will benefit.

No, I do not think that is controlling in any way. It would just make the world operate on a balanced playing field. Darth Vader™ would probably make the following support statements:

The militaries should all be repainted to fly the U.N. banner initially and then a new banner created for Earth by that body. There should still be representation by the old countries in the U.N. much like as in our Senate and House. Not too much democracy though. Over-governance is exactly the thing that inhibits world progression. All the nations who chose not to participate should be bombed the fuck out of. Note: If you live in a country that has a history of rebelling against the larger powers, you should probably leave. We send 500,000 troops with massive air support and really large tanks into say Cuba and Iraq concentrated on the singular task of finding and killing or imprisoning the motherfuckers who used to lead those countries and then we horsewhip the rest of their militaries into shape. That's all there is to it. What the hell is so hard about that?

A leader should be chosen from among those who have worked to establish peace within their personal lives. This person could come from any country including the impoverished. They should still be a strong leader though as they will inevitably be responsible for further public contact with all alien species. They will also have to request funds and support for parts of the world that are not up to par with the technologies and advances in say health care that are available to make better our lives. That person should strive to preserve monuments and to erect new ones in tribute to the spirit of accomplishment and human invention and ingenuity (but no new monuments in Israel). Politics needs to have nothing to do with a world leader. What would that person be politicking for? There would be no legitimate reason for that person to have any bias or any malice in their hearts toward any sect of persons. Current world leaders should not even be made eligible. There would be too much motive for personal greed. The person who was awarded such a position should not even be given monetary reward or salary. They and their family should just be taken care of simple as that. If you take wealth out of the equation, you take out most of the possible motivation for greed and greedy actions.

Remember, I am writing here about a future PLANETARY leader that makes planetary ecological and representational decisions, not about conquest or the merging of nations and the destruction of culture.

There should be no one house of governance within the world but rather several places which the chosen leader and the U.N. should have to visit and hold meetings within. This eliminates the thought of favoritism and promotes understanding. Imagine what would happen if a world meeting were made to take place in the deserts of India and then in a downtrodden town in Ecuador. Two months later it would be in Ireland and then back to Hiroshima. Without armchair, air conditioned, fat, stinky old ass-holes with bad hair in a senate atmosphere very cool and impressive things would happen I could assure you. For people to be fair and unbiased on the whole, they must be placed in the midst of the people they represent.

The new world nation would produce faster and better space exploration methods and vehicles. Cooperation would end most poverty. Cities would get cleaned up, and the entertainment industry would have a much broader scope with which to work. Education levels would soar without international boundaries. Finally, and my personal favorite, there would be much more space for us all to spread out in and not bother each other so much. Transportation will improve and make living on top of each other unnecessary.

IT IS DONE

Recently I speculated that since the inception of the Euro that there were forces at work to do this in other parts of the world. Turns out I was right. President G.W. Bush and the leaders of Canada and Mexico have already signed an agreement that would create the Amero-dollar. _It's already done baby!_ You don't have a choice. Regionally there will be two other mass economic unions. One I believe is for India, the Ukrainian breakaway countries and parts of Africa and I think the other is for the Asian communities. I will admit to being a little foggy on those two right now. Once those systems are in place, the plan is to give them several years or decades to work out the kinks and then combine the 4 regions into 1. Amazing huh?

So the world will not be conquered through military force, but through a system of commerce. It is a little scary. The only crooked part of the whole deal is in the printing of the money and in the banking systems as it pertains to various national debts.

Explanation: in the United States our treasury system is not owned or even regulated by the Government. No lie! It began as a conglomeration of about 5 wealthy banking clans that agreed to print the same type of money in the early 1900's and then they strong-armed the smaller banks into submission. This currency is printed by the new treasury and essentially lent to the people of America. The treasury is making money in the form of interest paid back on every dollar that it prints. So much of our national debt essentially does not really exist. It continues to be put in the pockets of these few families and their descendents. If the new world government claims Eminent Domain over the FED and prints its own new world money then we just tell the treasury families to go fuck themselves. This plan can work. No more interest accrued national debt! As you will read later, it doesn't make any sense for a government to owe money to someone else. They just take what they need anyway.

CRIME IN GENERAL

Now the fact of the matter is that anyone who does not believe in capital punishment is just a big old stanky pussy (pardon the term). By all means, let the punishment fit the crime. There is too much crime all over the world, and that directly attributes to the fact that many people are too afraid to enjoy traveling to countries like Columbia or Croatia. Most of the people there are extremely friendly.

In fact I don't think the philosophy of cutting of the hands of a thief is all that bad. The only instance that I would even support the claims of a thief would be if they had stolen only enough food for them to survive on, but as you already know that would not be an issue under my free basic staples program.

Theft is actually very upsetting to everyone because it always seems to happen to the innocent at a bad time. Not that there is ever a good time, just that it seems to make life more all around "shitty". There's not much that you can do about it either, but there is something you can say. Almost everyone knows someone who is a hoodlum and a thief. If the circumstance exists that you and the thief both know what has been done to obtain the merchandise, by continuing to be a part of their lives and by keeping conversation with them you unwittingly are saying "it's all good!" You are non-verbally communicating that you inherently approve of the behavior or you would in fact say something. That makes you a third-party accessory in my book. Now what are the odds that we all know someone who has committed theft? Pretty high. I had a struggle with this in my past as my ex-father-in-law and my ex-wife are both massive thieves. (They are not going to appreciate reading this but it's true.) All I am asking is for you to be consciously aware of the rotten person you might be and try to change it when the opportunity comes around again. I marked the calendar with a big X on the last day that I stole something, which was a 1 gallon fuel embellishment from a previous employer. It made me feel better to put it down on paper and it did the job of reminding me to change. I haven't taken anything again since that day.

RETRIBUTION

"Do unto others, as you would have them do unto you" or something to that effect. People get away with theft and all manner of other crimes because we really don't hit criminals where it hurts. Jail time is an inconvenience, but it's not the same as retribution offered up because it is the right thing to do.

Personal Retribution is the term that I would use to describe this type of veneration that I feel the victims of crimes should receive. My theory is that once apprehended and convicted, all the personal property or holdings of the assailant shall be given to the victim or the victim's family, to do with as they choose. They can keep them, sell them, light them on fire or donate them to another continent. This would include land and homes, vehicles, monetary gatherings, personal affects and record collections.

If a person has a reasonable doubt that another person has taken any article of property from their premises, the accused should be subject to an immediate search of their premises, and automobile. We have a term for this now called "Reasonable Doubt". Should that search turn up the missing article an equal and greater retribution may take place at the discretion of the person who suffered the original loss. If you're not guilty you shouldn't get bent out of shape by the accusation. When you are cleared, your accuser would have to apologize publically (i.e. In the Newspaper) and bake cookies for you and a homeless shelter as a public service.

RAPE

Crime touches us more severely in the form of rape. The sex offender not only violates the victim's body but their psyche as well. The percentage of women who have suffered some form of sexual attack is not acceptable. I don't know any women who are strong enough to not let this affect them emotionally, and why shouldn't it. Your parents and family are affected even if they do not know about it. They do recognize your mood changes and often-explosive tones that begin to leak out, or maybe it's the lack of interest in doing anything that sparks their concern. Every subsequent male in this person's future then feels the results of the attack. They will always be hurt, concerned and want revenge on your behalf. That's just the way it is.

Some victims conceal it better than others, but it always results in either a lack of affection and trust for someone who has worked hard to gain it, or an unwillingness to even attempt a relationship. Some women erect a wall so great that it would take Batman's grappling gun to overcome. They are so afraid of being hurt now on any level that it is worth it to them to shut out the entire world. This is a crime in itself as some of these women are truly beautiful people all the way through and they have an amazing capacity to love. Very often it can only be expressed from that moment on to a pet. The only way to even feel better is first through revenge and then followed by clean living and developing a close relationship with God.

So why should we let a rapist get a free ride in jail for just a few years? What do you think of these punishment standards? Prisoners having been convicted of rape will receive without condition or exception by a judge;

1. Mandatory life term of 10 years incarceration.
2. A brutal violation of their person in the same manner of the crime committed, to be administered by prison

guards with a nightstick or similar club dipped in chili pepper sauce in the rectum on the anniversary of the crime for the duration of their 10-year sentence.

3. Video footage should be made available to the victim and for public viewing to teach future generations a sterner lesson.

4. The rule of Personal Retribution shall apply.

Hate crimes and other attacks resulting from jealousy, misinformation, or blatant stupidity are also unacceptable. Let's deal with hate crimes first. I simply do not understand what it is that a bigot sees in others as being different or less perfect from them. In almost every case the minority is far superior to their attacker in some way. As a rule, physical and mental prowess is something that Anglo people are generally far behind the rest of the world in. What is it going to take to make these people realize that we are all human and all brothers? There are far greater things to be concerned with than this. When will we recognize all life as being worthy and having rights? Goats and baby sheep in the fields have rights too you know. There's my little PETA plug...just for my brother Shane who is a major activist.

The punishment for hate crimes should be as radical as it can get. Let the criminals be subject to the same ridicules as are mentioned for rape, but let them be carried out by the hand of a person of the same race, in areas populated by the race of people they persecuted. *Humiliation* is the key.

CAPITOL PUNISHMENT

Now we just don't even need inmates who have committed murder. We don't need their stupid appeals either. If you think you want them alive, let them live in your house. I'm sure you'll play lots of games and have wonderful picnics together. They obviously didn't learn the lesson in this life so let them move on to the next, where they get to keep on trying and keep on being punished until they get it right. If an individual brings him or herself to commit a murder than we owe it to ourselves to torture that person unmercifully until they are dead. None of this "soft killing" garbage either. By this I mean mostly lethal injection but the gas chamber is pretty lame as well. Bring out the bull-whips, let insects eat them alive, pour acid on open wounds, feed them plenty of laxatives, break all of their finger and toe nails and make them swallow Listerine. I think I like the bugs and creepy little animals best. It puts distance between the executioner and the recipient.

THE RACKS

I would like to know who decided to get rid of punishing our criminals in public. I suppose this goes back to the hanging and burning days, but we didn't have to take it out of view altogether. They needed a marketing genius back then. Public humiliation is one of the most damaging things you can do to a criminal. Did I already mention that? Not only did they get caught, but now everyone can taunt and laugh at them. I think that a sign should be posted a safe distance from the prisoner explaining what their crime was and the manner in which they were caught. That way the public has some material to use as ridicule, especially if a stupid mistake was made. Rotten vegetables should not only be allowed, but also made available. These could be donated by the local food banks that always have some waste whether it is melons, lettuce, bananas, or tomatoes. This could also serve as a legitimate write off for grocery stores and suppliers to donate to the food bank.

Children should be allowed to view this from a distance and from behind a sound barrier such as a Plexiglas wall. There will undoubtedly be some verbal abuse flying, and our children learn this soon enough. We can have a teacher or tour guide explain what is going on. At just the right age, just before it becomes funny to them and is still a little frightening, a deep impression will be made and thus with a little fear of God and some respect for the consequences we will have a lot less future crime.

GRAFFITI and LITTER

The award for the best looking city in the nation has to go to the Metro-Phoenix area. Phoenix kicks ass in terms of being a beautiful place to live. Too damn smoggy now though and the urban sprawl got out of control in the late 90's. It has become like L.A. in that respect. Often called and awarded the "Best Run City in the World", it does do an exceptional job of keeping its roadways clean. They do this through various sponsorship programs (road sign with name or company logo) and by utilizing the ever-popular chain gangs. The inter-city freeways are even lined with flowers and decorative pots. It is a superior effort on the part of the city maintenance staff. If you've never been there, you don't how nice your city could look.

Now as for graffiti, does anybody really like seeing gang writing? Does gang writing turn you on? Does it make you want to pull your car over and masturbate while you look at the pretty art? No, I didn't think so. If someone you know typically signs their gay initials on the bathroom hand dryer, tell them out loud what a loser they are. If they don't hear it from a friend then it means nothing from an authority! Make sure you let them also know that graffiti is an onset characteristic of becoming a gay pedophile. This should adequately convey your disgust.

Littering is against the law. At least in America this is a fact. In most parts of the country it is punishable with up to a $500 fine and possible jail time. So why then do we do it? I am going to hazard a guess and say that only 1 in 1,000 people in America today do not litter in some form. I fear it may be higher than that. Why would you want to live in a city or place with trash on the side of the roads?

Cigarette butts are of course the worst, and I say that without malice toward the people that smoke. *As a group you are some lazy sons-of-bitches.* Cigarette butts look terrible laying everywhere. Double punishment for you people just because the item is small and it takes a lot of time to clean up.

Here is what I want. The power authorized by the ATF (Bureau of Alcohol, Tobacco & Firearms) to pull people over, bind them with ankle cuffs and let them start cleaning within a 100-foot radius of where their trash landed. The disruption of their otherwise valuable time combined with the degradation of their personal character as others go by and laugh and the stiff fine will help curb that behavior. Really I want to be an enforcer type Federal Field Marshall or something to that effect. Put me in charge man! We'll have a new definition of Marshal Law.

FIGHTING

There is a time when every man just feels the need to get in a good fight. There is nothing wrong with that but most of the time we do go to jail. You probably wouldn't think that I would support this kind of behavior; however I do to a point. It's perfectly natural. We're just being protective and territorial. It's nothing an animal wouldn't do. I want to fight people all the time, I just don't want to go to jail for it.

I think fighting should be legal and encouraged. Just as long as before you start, the participants should have the presence of mind to clear the area of children and agree not to use any weapons or friends. When one person is sufficiently broken or battered, then it's over. No harm done and no consequences as long as nobody dies. If you break somebody's tooth you would have to pay for that on the principle of basic human rights. People with nice teeth worked hard for those. Punch them somewhere else. There are plenty of options. Noses will even heal, but teeth don't. Testicles aren't cool either. *Would a lion bite you in the testicles during a fight? Even if the lion was losing, I doubt it.*

TERRORISM

No book written or distributed after September 11, 2001 would be complete without a personal insert about the incidences of that day. While my condolences of course go out to the families who suffered losses in the tragedy, there are two major concerns that stick out in my mind.

One: They were the largest towers in the world at one time, so where was their protection. They were an obvious target from day one. Care to guess what I would have done? Ok, there should have been a few National Guardsmen stationed on the roof at all times with a battery of missiles so that any deviance from any flight plan would have been met with a halting blow. Not to be cruel, but the strike planes are empowered to shoot down commercial airliners now, so why not in defense before something devastating happens? The same basic structure of defense holds true for Washington D.C. and every other major target. That one was basic idea and it should have been implemented a long time ago.

Two: As it pertains to terrorism, yes the act is fanatical, but it isn't really about a show of force. Being a terrorist from the psychological standpoint is more about making your personal mark in history. The terrorist M.O. is such that they want to feel important. Many of the lackeys that carry out the work do not have the sense of personal worth or clarity of thought to determine right from wrong in the face of a strong, wealthy and thus persuasive leader. They just want to take what they can, go out with a bang and know that they stood for something and made an impact on the world, even if it was for somebody else's dream.

As for the fanatical leaders themselves, it takes a hell of a lot of money and time to pull off a campaign of that magnitude. With some superior marketing efforts that money that could have been put to better uses while ensuring their future fame and notoriety. Do you know how much all-virgin monkey porn you could make with that kind of money? It would just be stupid!

They could still have affected a change in the lives of people. For example; it has been said that the accused organization for the tragedy on 9/11/01 is bankrolled to the sum of 300 million dollars U.S. Just think of all the things you could do with that money to affect change in the world. As of this date our largest Powerball jackpot was only some 12 million short of that amount and every American dreamed of the things they could do to live in infamy forever. It is a pity really that more winners don't do something positive. They just take the money, run and hide. That is not what Spiderman would advocate. If Spiderman won the lottery, he would be responsible and giving! If I don't do it, someone and Warren Buffet needs to put together a website / 501c-3 called www.lotterywinners.org so that the world can make suggestions in an open format. I should be on the Board of Directors at least.

Anyway, the point is that many factories could have been opened along with several hundred restaurants and a theme park or two. Grants could be given for neighborhood improvements, or a nationwide urban renewal and cleanup project could be undertaken. Jobs would be created, the country in question would look better and the "would-be" terrorist goes down as a hero rather than a demon to millions.

Remember that one good deed and the sacrifice it takes to make it happen are worth all of the riches in the world.

One final thing about 9/11 and the conspiracy theories; yeah - we as a nation are pretty much blind. I'm gonna leave this as an open topic for you to do your own research. Start with Tower 7 that magically imploded but wasn't hit with anything. Look at the support struts in the 2 main towers that sure seemed to be pre-cut with concrete saws. Explosions occurring before the planes hit. Do the math! We have too much internal bad shit going on to be worried about much else. People are worried about getting assassinated if they talk. Really?

Since this is such a heated topic I will include that I personally believe that it was **BOTH** a terrorist job AND since we knew it was coming we had an inside job helping it to collapse for whatever reason.

People, you and I do not know the whole story. We probably never will. There is bad shit constantly in play on both sides. It is not unfathomable to think that it could have happened this way. I am not saying we collaborated with the terrorists, merely suggesting that someone, somewhere in the Bush administration took advantage of an existing situation to further another cause.

Did I mention that I am running for President in every future election until I die?

Now, go back to page 87 and read this chapter again, right now since I am 100% sure that you did not grasp everything correctly. Thank you.

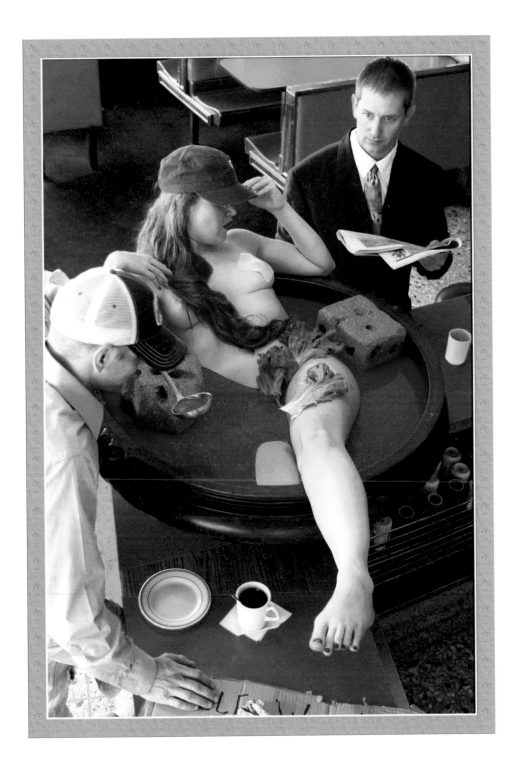

Tomato Girl Soup

I am so proud of this shot. It took a year to set it up.

A bleak portrait depicting the hopelessness of everyday modern work life and the means with which we sustain ourselves. The executive pictured is in a standard café and not in an expensive luncheonette setting. This is representative of the average white collar worker who is not really at all impressed with the corporate bull shit of the executive world. The soup represents the physical nourishment that his body requires and is very often lacking. The girl coming out of the soup is the incarnation of the one thing that refreshes his mind and empowers him to carry on the façade for his co-workers for the rest of the workday. You will note that hot coffee is being served instead of the booze traditionally associated with naked women. That is because this place is necessary in his mind and he is not there for mere entertainment.

Exactly the same is true for the homeless vet except that his general disregard is for everything else. He at least has a Miller Lite ball cap. He would consider adding booze to the cauldron except for that all the patrons have to share this one delicious bowl and someone else might not like his flavor of MD 20/20.

Date Taken: August 2009

Location: Tom's Diner, on Colfax in Denver, CO

Model: You have to pay her a LOT to find out!

Concept By: Parrish Douglas

Photo Taken By: Parrish Douglas

ECONOMY

CHAPTER V

So our economy sucks a dirty unleavened donkey ass. Yes...yes it does. Drink 'till it gets better and invest in booze companies. You can blame the past administrations if you want to, but it's a moot point. Almost every country is in the same boat. I am arguing that we need to not be such greedy bastards and the problem will iron itself out. More on that in a moment.

My brother Roderick tells me that I am a Communist and that I skew Nazi in my economical views. That's almost correct. He hates this chapter and even stopped reading he got so mad. People get visibly upset when I express that we should control the birth rate until we whittle down the population to only the useful people. Here is parable is for you to understand socialism a little better. A man in Poland told me this; "Communism works very well for the people who draw the right number. If you only have to work from 10 to 2 and you play the flute, then you like it. If your job is picking up trash for 12 hours then it's not so good." I'm just bitter 'cause in my earlier life I drew the losing number so I want everyone else to suffer the same fate as a young person. At the very least though, most people under that structure got paid the same. Maybe not fairly; but the equal to each other.

Now then, the unemployment rate of the great depression was over 10% and according to the Onion periodical out of Boulder, CO-Dec. '09 the **labor availability rate** is at 10.2% so fuck yeah we're in a depression. Stop dancing around the point call it what it is.

It is a sad state of affairs in this country that the income poverty level for a family of four is about $19,000 / year. I can tell you that in reality, for single people to be able to have their own living space, and to enjoy life, $19,000 is the bare minimum one can get by on. I know this because I was a professional at getting things for free for a long time. Had I not been able to do so, I would have been forced to move back in with my parents. This doesn't mean that I am lazy and cannot find a good job. I believe everyone wants to work at something that makes him or her happy. What it does mean is that things are too hard today for businesses to survive and pay their employees a decent wage. Remember when half the population was forced to invade peoples homes by doing telemarketing because it was the only easy to get, good paying job? What a nightmare those days were.

As a side note, I'll bet the joker who developed telemarketing has never made a cold hard sales call to a _cranky person who sternly voices their opinions_ in his or her whole life. That person was only a strategist. It is a hard thing to be constantly yelled at and rejected.

WAGES

What is the thinking behind the following theory? "Let's raise the minimum wage so that we can charge more for everything." It doesn't make any sense but that's what happens. First we raise the minimum wage to a whopping $5.25 (or whatever, it's not enough to even be worth remembering), and then Milk goes up to $3 a gallon and a movie ticket is now at $9.50 in a small city. I remember when I could say, "Those poor people in New York City have to pay $7 to see a show." What is the point of raising prices? Someone's a greedy son-of-a-bitch. A few someone's in fact.

112

I propose that a new law be put into affect that any company or corporation which _nets_ free and clear more than $10,000,000 (ten million) dollars in a year must pay every full time employee a salary of at least $30,000 per year. I know that this must seem absurd to those of you who run such companies but let's take a moment to explore this. I would also like to propose that no person making a gross wage of less than $30,000 be made to pay any taxes at all. It's just not a lot of money. Still at $30,000 you are just getting by, but it would make a little difference if you got to use the full wad.

If you doubt what I am saying right now, go to any McDonalds and ask the food prep staff if they would like a 100% raise. Are you beginning to see the point yet?

What builds a thriving economy in any situation you can think of is the spending of currency on goods and services. Now then, bearing in mind that it is 2010 and the average full time worker at a retail or service industry job is earning between $24k - $30k pre-tax, I think a pay increase of nearly 30% would make me pretty damn happy and a lot more productive. Ok, so this would now mean that a family of four would have a gross/net income (same thing at that pay level) of at least $60,000 if both parents worked full time, which in most parts of America they do. Now assume that the cost of child care did not go through the roof (as I'm proposing it should not) as well as the cost for food, transportation, education, and housing. Here's the future you will witness. Everyone will have nice spacious homes, there won't be many bad neighborhoods at all, everyone could afford to get a college education, we'd be well fed and clothed, and in short _we'll spend the money!_

Drastically changing the base platform in our society will result in more business being transacted and more jobs being created. We could finally achieve a thriving economy not on the verge of collapse.   The real trick is that we have to be decent human beings and not cheap bastards.

One more argument that I would like to make is that we don't even need a stock exchange. *Do you realize that 98% of the stock market system is comprised of people who have no life skills other than math and corruption, which is more of a loathsome trait and less of an actual skill.* They are just afraid to get their hands dirty and do some honest labor, so they created the stock exchange system. IT DOESN'T DO ANYTHING PEOPLE! <u>We don't absolutely need it to survive.</u> There are some analysts out there right now saying "shit he figured it out. Now we're going to have to raise a stink and do counter-interviews on CNN and talk radio."

TAXES

For those of you who happen to be tax attorneys or CPA's, just skip this part. You're not included in the nightmare of confusion with the rest of us.

A person never knows if their employer will take out enough for taxes or not, regardless of which numbers you claim on your w-4 forms. Taxation remains something of a mystery to me. Sure I understand the basic principles of money to help run the government, but none of these reasons for taxing do the general population a fat wad of visible good.   We see some road maintenance and improvements, some new parks every now and then, but I think we'd all like to know where the rest of it is going.

Appointed offices, like the President, Senators, Judges and other heads of state should just be provided for. Do we really have to give them a salary?   Can't we just give them official U.S. diplomatic vouchers that they can give to the retailers at which they shop? Then the retailers can use them as a tax write-off at the end of the year. ← *That last idea right there is fucking brilliance in action! I came up with that all on my own!*

By doing this then we don't have to worry about them giving themselves raises. When they are forced to leave office they should be given a severance package and reintroduced into the workforce like everyone else. I say give them jobs at Dillard's or a bakery or something not quite at the bottom but certainly at the median wage that the rest of the country is living on at the time. I also think that we should make it illegal for them to try to skip out of such a civic duty and reintroduction program unless they are already at retirement age.

It seems to the working class people of this country that the government already does take whatever it wants. Likewise it seems that our tax money is going into someone's pocket. I can say this because despite being cool I am also still working class.

Keep in mind what I said earlier about the $30,000 minimum taxable limit. From there the next raise your employer would have to give you would be at least $10,000 to offset the fact that you would now be taxed. $6,000 of that 10k would go to the government leaving you with really just an average raise. That's not an unheard of raise for a company to give you if they really value your employ.

I propose that they take a flat rate and an easy one to calculate; say 10% of our total gross income and then leave us alone. No more filing taxes or reporting to the IRS because we could close down that agency down, or at least down size it to a regulatory agency. Every person should still check the numbers to make sure that 10% and only 10% exactly is ever taken out. There are just too many people and too many headaches for us to have to deal with such an *ARCHAIC* system as taxation and the reporting thereof.

Social Security and welfare should get 1% each that is derived out of the 10% mentioned above. No more, no less. If we are all working on the $30,000 minimum wage program of mine, and you still aren't smart enough to save something for your own future then that's just too bad. Kids are there to support you. Why did you have kids again? Oh yeah, that chapter full of insults comes later.

By the way, if a person wants their Social Security and welfare money before they turn 65, we should just let them have it. Sometimes a person just wants to be lazy and sometimes people treat their bodies so harshly that they know they are not going to make it to be old anyway. I don't care and neither should the government but when you slice of the pie is gone, then it's gone. Good luck to you after that.

.95 .98 and .99

You're not fooling me by pricing a car at $19,999.99 ok? That's 20 thousand dollars you fuckers. When you search for a home you don't choose one that is priced at $299,999 over one that is $300k. Gas prices are the same way too. It just pisses me off that the government can't make a no bull-shit price law. You don't get a hotel room for $99. It's a $100 alright. Let's just live in the real fucking world for 2 seconds. How much did you pay for this book? I hope and pray that it was right on the dollar. It will be hard for me and the publishers to enforce this because every state has different taxation levels. 6% or 7.5% or 0% if you live in Texas or Oregon I think. At least you will know that we made the effort. Constantly annoying to this writer and insulting to my intelligence are the pricing strategies of those who sell retail goods. Ranging from clothes to gas and sometimes food, the item is marked as near to the next highest amount as possible. I understand the theory is that we will look at the first few larger numbers and decide then if that product fits into our expenditures range. I think this is cruel to be honest. Don't we have enough to think about without having to round up the price of every purchase? In the case of major purchases such as large televisions, cars, and homes, this could cause a nice credit problem to someone who is not paying attention. (Slimy sales tactics do not help either.)

As a note to retailers; for the sake of convenience I ask that you do the a-fore mentioned rounding for us. If you really want to impress your customers, figure the tax into the prices you mark on your shelves or billboards. To add another step, I personally would manipulate this after tax figure to equal the nearest dollar, .50 or.10 cent marks. I don't like carrying change and I'll bet that I'm not the only one. We have too much other crap in our pockets or purses to dig for. On the male side, you can't carry change if you're wearing dress slacks. It doesn't stay quiet. Having to hold it in place while you walk so you don't sound cheap is not cool. You just end up throwing at somebody.

WASTE

We are living now in a time where nearly everything is recyclable yet we continue to purchase one use items and things that will regularly break down. The term for this is "planned obsolesce". Newspapers, magazines, are one example. Let me explain. Reading material in the future of America will all be available on computer. Right now I hope that ½ of you are reading this in an EBook format! Most of it is now but you just have to subscribe to someone's Internet service. I suppose I should include the figures of how many trees get the ax every year for this but we all know its something ridiculous like 400 acres per day or more. Laptop computers are becoming readily available and if we follow my plan to pay every full time worker $30,000 I think people will be happy to invest in something that takes the clutter from their lives. I don't own shit. I am a total minimalist and I relish in the freedom and peace of mind that it brings.

There is an appeal to hard copy books though. They feel good in your hands. I insisted on making this available for download and hopefully soon I can make it for audio books so you can hear the disgruntled tone in my voice. The point that I make and that any intelligent person cannot refute is that a book is for many a refuge in a way that a current events periodical is not.

The amount of waste that we create as a society is incredible. Why do we do this? Well because if we didn't make useless crap then a lot of people would be out of a job but we don't really need so much junk or even so many choices within the junk categories. I choose to believe in something that is a contradiction to what we all learn as children: that is a returh to simplicity through technology.

No, I don't believe in recycling and I don't care about that one fish that got his head stuck in a plastic 6 pack can holder. We build our own neighborhoods on landfills. Do you realize the kind of shit that goes into a landfill? That could be under your house but now you're supposed to care about the planet for future generations. I'm gonna be dead. You're gonna be dead. If God reclaims the Earth in 2016 we're all gonna be dead and God has the power to make the landfills disappear and turn into beautiful lakes. If God makes a beautiful 3-eyed fish that's His business. I like mutations. Ever since I was a kid I wanted to be an X-man!

REAL ESTATE and MORTGAGE

Everyone and their moms think they are qualified to sell real estate or fix/flip homes. It's just not so. "You fuckers" (author shakes his head and rubs temples). In fact I wish about ¾ of the cum-stain agents out there would quit. (By that I mean that you should never have been born) They are just terrible and have almost no people skills. I am really including this little section just because I happen to be an Independent Employing Broker as one of my side ventures. I am an AWESOME agent and that's exactly why I don't see many deals. The pool is too clouded with liars for you to find the good ones. Almost 100% of both RE and Mortgage agents don't give a damn about what you want or what you think.

I see far too many people as potential clients who are not qualified but they ask me for advice and want free help. It's just like asking a person for relationship advice that you have no intention of following. Don't do it. Please refrain from being a pain in the ass looky-loo if you know damn well that you're not qualified and you have no cash. Oh yeah, we call you names as soon as you walk out the door.

The days of "No Money Down" come and go but for the most part they stay gone for long periods of time. Don't listen to the lies. Don't believe the lies. You have to put your act together before you go looking for a house. I'm sorry. That's just how it is and anyone who disagrees with this statement is really just a third rate agent not worth their own weight in salt. You want to waste your time with pretenders, be my guest.

By the way, the only difference between a REALTOR and a Real Estate Agent is that people have to pay a lot of extra fees to be a member of the National Association of REALTORS. You can call NAR with some low level support questions but that's about it. Their website sucks hairy balls and it's not even run internally. It is a cluttered mess that they farm out to another website company that has nothing to do with real estate. Furthermore, the whole notion of you as a buyer looking for your own home online just undermines the whole industry and is putting people out of jobs. You should be looking online for an agent that you like and that you might enjoy spending some time with. Let us do our jobs please. We let you do yours right?

Here's the quick etiquette lesson for you qualified potential homebuyers. This mostly applies to young people because if you have gone through the process you should already know this. In most states an agent doesn't like taking you around to see properties until after they have two things from you. A valid letter of financial qualifications and an <u>Exclusive Right to Buy</u> contract that pretty much says you agree to not stab them in the back and use another agent after they have spent a bunch of time with you.

One last thing; foreclosures, short sales and investment properties take a lot more knowledge, time and money than most people care to admit. I flat out refuse to tell you how to do it. Carlton Sheets is a little bitch. All I am going to do is complain about all the infomercials and print advertisements and fucking lawn signs you see on the subject. "Become a millionaire in real estate". "Make CEO income from home". Those people are massive bloody douche-bag liars. I don't even have to be out on a limb to proclaim that. Just forget you ever heard the term foreclosure unless you have a LOT of cash in your pocket right now. Short sale really means "long sale" 'cause it takes so much fuckin' time. Understand? Are we good?

Oh, I earn that 2.8 or 3.2% from a RE deal and I hate the practice of rebating to the buyer or seller. You can't afford it and you need my money back, really?

I also am obligated to cover mortgage brokers since they are primarily the slime of the earth. Not all of you are now, but you <u>all</u> were very shifty at one time. Admit it. There are too many ways to hide money and get paid as much as 8 points on the back end of a deal. Even if your relative tells you they are giving you a deal, what they are really giving you is a steaming turd line. No mortgage broker ever works for free. That's fine. You earn your money too. I just don't agree with you lying to people and trying to hide it in several different parts of the deal. Your brother or your uncle absolutely did not do your deal for free. No fucking way in the fires of hell. I will bet you anything on the planet Earth that is mine to bet with. Now you pretty much have to get a mortgage from somewhere so I'm not complaining about that. Again, I am just saying watch out for hidden points. You have a right to know. The whole process is just so aggravating and time consuming that we just want it to be over quickly. If you verbalize your desperation at any point, you just opened up the gates of your financial ass to be raped by a white collar paper pushing rape artist.

Sorry guys and gals in the industry. You know I'm right. Don't cry because I just called you out, just be on the up and up with your clients. Tell them right up front "*I am going to make $10,000 on your deal and that's what I require to get it done. Do we have an agreement?*"

GREAT FOOD and FREE FOOD

Later on down the road in the chapter about sex, I will reaffirm what I am saying here. Everything is better when you make noises. That could include belching; however I am referring to intended verbalizations much like sex noises. It's a shame that more people aren't on board with this thinking. If you don't like to hear others make noises then you're too anal and you're eating the wrong things. This really does say a lot about your personal lives as well. "I'll have what she's having!" Remember that line from *When Harry Met Sally*? If you don't enjoy your food I bet you have a really lame sex life. Lame by my standards anyway.

I believe that hunger is one of the worst fates to befall anyone. Perhaps it affects me more than others. I get weak, dizzy, and impatient on a regular basis. Fortunately I know and listen to the early signs my body gives me. For some eating is a disease. For others it is the opposite. We live in a society where it is totally unnecessary for anyone to go without.

All the human dietary staples should be made free of charge and readily available to the public. 2 MORE points for Communism!

I know this one is pretty far out there. I am talking about milk, bread, cheese (the good stuff is ungodly expensive), bland cereals, and basic fruits-vegetables. Eggs are a maybe only because if you are a breakfast whore like me, then you could scam the system and get every meal for virtually free. That's not the goal, so we have to regulate eggs and good tasting cereal.

Now as with everything today there are many varieties of all of these things. Of course not all of them should be free. The rich can still pay for goat cheese. I'm talking about the pasty American singles version that the creative cook can use in a variety of ways. I'm talking about regular loaves of sliced bread, plain old round head (filling but no nutritional value) lettuce, normal sized tomatoes, bananas which go to waste anyway, a very cheap wheat-grain-or-corn based cereal (maybe one chocolate variety), and milk. You get the idea. Everything that is exclusive, which is made to make you feel special, you should still pay for. I only want to eliminate hunger for poor people, of which I was definitely once one. I disguised it well and many people never knew, but I was still hungry.

MEDICAL CARE

All of this should be free and fast. This is one area where persons who find themselves unemployed from restructuring of one program would always be able to find work. Communism isn't all bad in these respects. How many people can you honestly name right now that badly need to go to the dentist? How many people have big, nasty warts and other shit growing off their faces? There are even more out there that have rashes, infections and cuts or bruises that won't get treated because they can't afford the $150 doctor visit, which by the way rarely does anything for anybody. Can we make it a law that doctors have to do something when you go to see them? People want some damn medicine. Things that end in the suffix "-cillin". Nobody gives a rat's ass about addiction to those drugs or a rising tolerance level. That's a fat load of crap that the medical community gives us and if you are stupid enough to take "-cillin" based drugs all the time for every little ailment then you Sir or Ma'am are a jackass and deserve to keep your rash. We can fix many health problems for animals without specialists or repeat visits so why not enable ourselves?

Reduce the costs of medicines too. It's not like were going to break the backs of pharmaceutical companies. We just shouldn't have to pay $35-60 for a basic prescription. It's a little tiny pill or some damn cream for God's sake. Health Care and Drug cost mark-ups just piss me off. I could go on and on about how non-surgical doctors should be limited to a $100,000/year salary and in fact I probably will later on.

EDUCATION

Much like medical care this should be completely free to anyone who wants one. Norway has an awesome system AND a negative birth rate. Never mind their 60% tax rate. I'll figure out a way around that in time.   Let's be serious.   No one likes an uneducated fool. Not everyone cares about higher education and that's fine. Some very wonderful people I know never went to college a day in their lives. How in the hell did they get good jobs? Especially in my former industry of radio broadcasting, one does not have to have an ounce of talent, only and Uncle or friend in the business. <u>I fully intend to make a connection and take somebody's job On-The-Air while out doing interviews and signings for this book.</u>

I have thoughts about early education strategies as well as middle and high school theories.   These are found primarily in the reproduction chapter and most of you will probably not like them at first. If you do not then once again I tell you that you have closed your mind.

INSURANCE

We need insurance to protect us from the fraud and scandals of insurance companies. Deductibles? What kind of weird crock of shit is this? Let's be real. Isn't the reason we pay our premiums in the first place, so that in the event that were ripped off or in an accident, we don't have to pay a dime for anything?

<u>Life Insurance</u> - Why do we pay so that others can get rich when we die? It should be called the Next-of-Kin fund.   This is potentially the biggest money making racket in the history of the world. My Father, God bless his soul had to sell insurance for 13 years to provide for us. I know it was hard and stressful. He should have written a book about how to successfully raise hell when you're a short man in the military -or- about creating the foundation for a 50 year marriage with 3 kids while you're out of

the country. *My father is a great man.* He had his first heart attack that nearly killed him during his Life Insurance sales tenure.

I just wrote a whole paragraph about how I hate to pay insurance premiums of any kind. I don't even have to explain myself do I? You completely hate them too!

Credit Card Insurance – This is a next level scam. I don't know of one single person who has ever been paid on this claim including for fraud insurance. I have been a victim of identity theft as have many people. Recovering your credit status shouldn't have to be your problem. Somebody else fucked up and the credit card companies allowed it, so yeah I think it is their duty to fix the problem without hassling you. Travel insurance in a foreign country may be the one legitimate service they provide.

So, to the point of all this; they want us to pay them $10 more per month for credit insurance. In the event that we die we don't have to pay them off. If we are dismembered we don't have to pay them off. Guess what, if we die then we won't care. If we become dismembered then we are going to sue the life out of everybody we can, then we'll have plenty of money to pay the damn thing off and we still won't care. If you're unemployed, destitute and living under a bridge then you don't care about your credit!

Auto Insurance - This scam is covered 2 chapters from now under Transportation.

Change of Life Direction Insurance - What about when we become laid off or more to the point when we just decide we have had enough of our current duties? We are in the year 2010. How many people just got laid off due to this depression? The national unemployment rate is at about 10%. So how about something useful like this? What about suicidal tendencies insurance? How about short term beach leave? What if we just can't take it anymore and go psychotic?

I am right the fuck there on the border. Sure it becomes a mental health issue and it needs to be proven that you are mentally unstable, but it could be done without a mountain of paperwork and 8 professional opinions. I certainly don't *want* to work anymore unless I am in radio or playing in a band. I would pay all year long for this kind of insurance but I guarantee I would cash it in every 3 years!

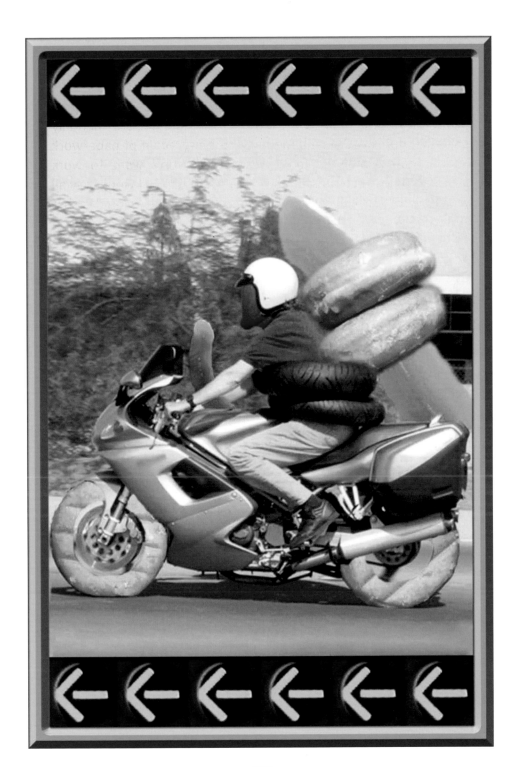

Spare Tire

I needed a photo here that was going to be so disturbing that it would stick in your mind forever. I think I succeeded. Now, whenever you see a green light you will be reminded of a giant green dildo sticking through some donuts and a retard on a motorcycle; but more importantly you will subconsciously remember to *STEP ON THE FUCKING GAS PEDAL IMMEDIATELY WHEN THE LIGHT TURNS FUCKING GREEN BECAUSE GREEN MEANS GO FAST RIGHT NOW YOU STUPID LAZY FUCK!!!*

I am sorry you have to see that but I really feel that shock value is necessary to "literally" drive home this point. If you're slow, get off the road. Go the fuck home and stay there forever. I really don't even want to see you on a bus because I hate busses. When we film the movie version of this book, I am pushing hard for a big destructive tank on the freeway that not only fires shells and leaves tread marks in the blacktop but I also want to run over the top of old people and kill them dead! I do actually need mental help, yes. This is the kind of shit I think about. You can't even fathom road rage on my level.

Big green cocks and donuts mean go fast. Whose idea was it to fuck an apple pie anyway? It's logistically no good. An average homemade pie is only 2.5" deep. That's not satisfying. Now fucking donuts; that's a perfectly normal reaction to a tasty hole.

Date Taken: Roughly 1997 Phoenix, AZ

Model: "Dick Face" I don't actually know this guy.

Photo and Art: Parrish Douglas

TRANSPORTATION

CHAPTER VI

Think you're a good driver? Ha, of course you do. The current state of transportation is something that enrages nearly every driver on the planet. Why can't I just go 90 through a school zone? Every one of us wishes that someone else would get out of our way. That is why this chapter is so vitally important. In it you will read about different schools of thought and the ways to combat the problems that we all seem to have. Decide for yourself when you are finished what category you fall into now and at what level you would like for your skills to become.

I'll tell you right now that I can tell that my own driving skills are slipping. I used to be just fucking phenomenal, Class AA+. I'm not really sure if age is catching up to me. It may be that the drugs I am on are slowing my reflex time. I suspect the latter, which is fine if it means being calm. I can still drive like a demon. I can drive you into the river, rest assured. I guess I'm just starting to wonder when the first big crash of my career will take place.

Everything else you do that pertains to moving your body; do it fast. Walk fast and tall. Walk with a purpose. If you happen to be in one of those moods where you just want to stroll around then please be kind and don't do it in the damn department store and for my sake please whack your children if they get in the way. I will body check a child that is in my path every time. Little bastards need to learn. Don't think that I won't check your kid when you're not looking 'cause if they are in my way they are about to get taken back to school.

ROAD CONSTRUCTION

Why is it that construction on our roads always seems to take so long? Have you ever thought that there should be a better way to make improvements? It occurs to me that a generally more viable solution to the current method of construction exists. Would that I were in charge of the department of roads, I think when the time came to make road upgrades, the logical thing to do would be to completely close the street in question.

Shut everything down, bring out the whole damned crew with all the equipment in the city, and work around the clock until it is finished. Can I say it any plainer than that? That's my plan and it shouldn't be done any other way. Think of all the money, time and energy that is wasted by closing off a section of road, tearing it up, rebuilding that section, creating a sub-road. It's not all that fun for the work crew either. I'm sure they would much rather go in and tear the hell out of the whole street and not even have to worry about damn pedestrians or getting hit themselves by cars. In stink-hole cities like Omaha where I used to live it once took them 9 years to finish a construction project on one section of highway. At one point it was so botched from all the re-routing that I think they just gave up and went home for a while. When I moved to Phoenix and saw these guys knocking out entire overpasses in less than six months I said, "Much better, that's the way!"

This method has several upsides and only one visible downside. Of course if the city were to close a road then nobody could use it until they were done. A bit of an inconvenience but when you compare it to the time frame of a completed project, then this pails as an argument. What all cities need to do is to appoint one guy who is a master planner and public relations expert. Whenever they want to do a project they should then do a splatter campaign all over the media (who should be strong armed if they don't cooperate). *"Stay **the fuck** off the freeway for* the next week. Ride the bus or carpool and it will be much better when were finished. Thank you for your attention in this matter."

* As it pertains to the sentence above, I like to place the expletives in the middle of the sentence after the action-directing verb such as "stay". This way if 90% of the emphasis of the sentence falls on a swear word, the person for whom the phrase is intended listens more and takes more of the message to heart. If I wrote "Stay off the fucking freeway", then the freeway (which is an inanimate object) becomes the focus of the sentence instead of YOU staying "the fuck" off of it, which is where the focus should be.

Finally as it pertains to construction, when we build cities why do we not just make the roads large to begin with? Shouldn't the planning and zone development people realize that there is an inherent value to wide open lanes that you can't put a price tag on? Every city that has anything to offer will eventually grow in the middle and have to expand or eventually sprawl. Just make the roads nice and big before any obstacles like homes get in the way.

Does this make sense to anyone but me? I hope so. I hope I'm not rambling on about things that don't make sense.

It's hard to be brilliant in our society. It's a very unrewarding career and we have a high rate of schizophrenia among ourselves. I'll tell you why this is. Most hyper-intelligent people have pensions for great conversation. When they can't find any then they turn inside. So for all the clinical psychiatrists who have patients like this, just put a few of them together with a couple hundred bucks and send them to a nudie bar. They'll be fine.

PUBLIC TRANSPORTATION

I am going to talk about this first and then work my way backwards into automobiles. That's how I think.

I like monorails. I think monorails are special. I think we should use them more. They go plenty fast, only have but 5 major stops, and they don't wait around for losers. If you can't get on board your wait is only 2 minutes because the next trains right behind. Look at how effectively they work for Disneyland. Walt had it going on at his place, and you know why it works so well, because he was a visionary. That and the fact that he owned everything so no one could tell him that it wouldn't work.

Now a monorail system is not going to work for everybody, and it's not supposed to. But it can legitimately move about 60% of any given population if the thing is designed right. Epicenter - downtown of course. Construct an arm to go to each major suburb or outlying city and an outer ring to alleviate even more congestion. Make the trains wide and long with plenty of seats. If the trains go fast you won't need any frills onboard. No Internet, no food, no beverages, no air-conditioning. Just move the thing *REALLY* fast! People don't pull out their laptops in the subway and they don't need to. Create nice big parking structures (which are free for all peoples for all of eternity), and the people will come. The people will use it. Hell it's my dream; I'll use it too.

Oh and by the way, there should be a **heavy** peace keeping contingent aboard every monorail car to kick the asses of any punk kids who get obnoxious! It should be a perfectly legal task force.

AIRPLANES

I want a massage chair that leans back 160° and massage footrest in first class. Why don't we have these already? It's the most uncomfortable thing ever to sit on a plane. I'd rather put my legs up in stirrups and have a damn baby. This is a no-brainer. Cost aside, tell me I am wrong on this one. Not one fuckin' person on the planet thinks airplane seats in coach are comfortable.

I also want to be able to have sex in my seat in first class. Then I want to cuddle up under a real blanket with some real pillows. I think we should have the option to skydive down to the landing platform and have someone deliver our baggage to us there. These are all non-negotiable points if I am going to pay that much money. I have never flown first class so far in my life. I am too cheap to justify doubling my ticket price just for only a kiss ass attendant. I want a really hot young chick to gently stoke my balls with her tongue for free and then feed me Crown Royal straight up when I ejaculate. I want to choose my movie from a large library. I want hanging hammocks from the ceiling so that I can stretch out for real and sleep when going overseas.

Most of all and I really mean this is the single most important mother-fucking rule for air travel: Get you fat bitch-ass off the plane FAST!!! Grab your damn bag and run off the plane. Sitting in the back of a hot nasty 737 is actually worse than rush hour traffic. What the hell is your problem? The gate attendants should have to check your dexterity and IQ before they let you bring any carry-on baggage because you're just going to be too damn slow. If I were a real air marshal I would just shoot you first with a .22 just to get your attention. Then we could take it outside where I would promptly stick and leave my steel toe boot directly in your ass while you're out there on the tarmac. Fuck, I hate you slow fuckers! I shouldn't even have got myself started on this one. Now I am mad and I am writing this at the airport. Must settle down...

My father suggested this one: Instead of de-icing the planes, which takes away an hour from everyone's life and uses a ton of resources why don't we just install something on the wings like a defroster for the back window of a car? They never break...ever, and they are so cheap to install. What a genius idea. Thanks Dad. We can do these things people! We have the technology! I will be the catalyst for change.

ALTERNATIVE POWER

Fossil fuels are obsolete. This is a fact. It is a wholly and as yet un-accepted fact, but a fact nonetheless. Can you let yourself believe that a culture capable of sending vehicles that must run indefinitely on solar power, to another planet like Mars, is incapable of making an automobile battery that can last for more than 80 minutes? Slow-ass busses continually spew toxic black fumes into the air by the cloud-full. I fuckin' choke on my own spit when that blows my way if I'm on a bike. How can that be better than a completely clean light rail or other _electric_ public transportation system?

The answer is very simple. Electric power is feasible. It is real and if we plan accordingly we have plenty of it. Greed is the only reason we still use gas. None of the greedy have an ounce of dignity or conviction or community vision, nor can they see that what they are doing is wrong.

Greed is a powerful thing. It is not one that I can say I have ever truly had to face, and for that I admit I am lucky. For those who have to face this beast though, it is not an acceptable excuse. Let me re-iterate. Being greedy in nature does not excuse one from seeking help and doing the right thing. It is a base and vulgar desire. There is not a greedy person in the world that has the right to consider themselves self an evolved being and/or worthy of controlling the transportation fate of the rest of us.

People are losing their jobs left and right as it is. You had to see this has been a long time coming. My plan isn't going to hurt anyone who isn't already hurting. We didn't need so many automobile choices in the first place. Now is the time to make a drastic change. Cute little hybrid cars aren't even close to the answer either. Scrap that idea completely. We need to go with something that is in a different direction and make a clean break from gas.

The car and even airplane industry is crawling at a pace that barely satisfies the citizens of the world. Did you know that an average size cruise ship moves approximately 8 INCHES on a gallon of gas?

MOVABLE WALKWAYS

Moveable walkways kick ass and there is not one person I know who is not instantly happier when they see one coming their way. If we are truly serious about cleaning up anything and offering the general public a viable means of transportation then I have the solution, and there is even a good way to govern the system while generating revenue too. The answer is movable walkways. In the future it will include suction tubes and teleporters. These things are so great for a number of reasons, the first of which is they take out and hospitalize all the stupid people who don't pay attention or tie their shoes. Secondly they entertain the fuck out of little children. Have you ever seen a child that wasn't completely fascinated by an escalator or walkway? I doubt it. Thirdly, they encourage mobility and exercise. If people are being moved, but they could walk or run and go faster than normal that is a total turn on. Of course they will do it and be healthier for it in the long run. We should even put them around public parks for the sake of fun.

So here is how to make the system work and be functional for all within acceptable parameters that will not make your city look too funky. These walkways should be thicker than those at the airports, about 4x's as wide. Let us say maybe 15 feet wide because we want to encourage mass use. They should generally be long so that people can traverse some distances. These will be especially effective in downtown areas where there are a lot of people who need to go perhaps only 4 blocks to lunch, but it is too long to walk and too short to drive. They should be raised above ground level so that the users will be revered as intelligent people and also so that they will have some scenery and a sense of continual motion, not having to stop for traffic or lights, 'cause stopping for cars does suck.

BIG BUSINESS

Here's how the whole thing needs to get paid for. Been to Las Vegas lately? I love it and it just keeps getting better. Everything that I just mentioned above has started to happen, only on a much smaller scale. At any rate there are walkways raised above major intersections on the strip. It looks as though some of the major casinos like the Caesars Palace "family" have fronted the bill for the construction, as the walkways resemble their hotels. It's not a bad idea to have big businesses in my future realm subsidize the building of the walkways, and then to have the cities pick up the tab for maintenance and power. They wouldn't have to spend as much fixing roads all the time. Sponsors would have the right to post classy, conforming signage where they see fit so that they get their much deserved recognition. Just as the major interstates are routed to certain tourist destinations, the walkways could be used to drive traffic to retailers and to promote product recall when a purchasing decision is made.

BUILDING THE BETTER BEAST

Now I don't really want to be giving all my brilliant ideas away to somebody else but that's pretty much the whole point of the book. I know a better way to do things and everybody just needs to listen to me. Payment for the ideas and transcription of such into forms that decision makers can understand will certainly be accepted though. Hire me on a consultancy basis.

It occurs to me that the point of producing different vehicles with different options is so that you can feel better and more prestigious than your neighbor. That is in fact reminiscent of some of the deadly sins listed later in the book. We are all the same on the inside with only slight variations of outward ugliness. We all have the same number of appendages though, and we all have the same internal organs and the same capacity to develop our minds and our awareness. This being said, if we have to have cars why would an automaker even want to offer some of their customers a more inferior vehicle than others? Wouldn't it make more sense to be known as the company that gives it all to everyone? I say let's load those babies up. Let's give them kick ass factory everything and do away with the concept of the base model. That just pisses people off anyway when they have to leave options off because you are charging extra for them. I am telling you that you would sell so damn many cars out of temptation that your freakin' head would pop off if you just put everything in them and only charged $1,000 over cost rather than $20,000 over cost. Don't be greedy man!

We also need U-turn signals. This is long overdue.

As long as I am on the subject, I might as well include something about warranties. Warranties are something like insurance in a way. If we are paying out the ass for a new car for the next 6 years of our lives don't you think we deserve to have everything fixed free of charge that goes wrong with your vehicle until were done paying for it? I do. Why do we need to pay extra for this? Just make a quality product.

Finally, do we really need the government to step in and tell the auto manufacturers that they have to produce more fuel efficient cars? Apparently, yes. WTF??? My 1985 Honda CRX got 40 mpg, no lie. What happened? Am I supposed to believe that we lost the technology on how to build those motors?

GOING TO THE CAR DEALERSHIP

Managers at dealerships are slimy brown ass-holes. Sure they have to make a living somehow, but could they at least exude a little dignity?

If you are one of these people here are a few tips that will help you save face in front of the world. First; if at any time someone you are dealing with wishes to leave the premises for whatever reason then you should let them go. Don't back peddle! Don't ask them any more insulting questions. If you have been on the level with your customers then it won't be an issue.

Second; when a customer chooses a vehicle that they like, tell them exactly what it costs to manufacturer the vehicle at the factory and then what it costs the dealer to purchase it (or the Invoice). What people want to know is how much of their money is going to both places not just the dealer. There is a preconceived notion that you are trying to rip us off, so just tell us "We make a flat $500 on every car we sell." OK! That's fair!

Third; never pass your customers off to anyone, even if it is the owner of the dealership. It is not appreciated and you instantly will turn the tide against you. What you are telling the customer is that you are incompetent as a salesperson and that all the time they have just spent with you has been wasted. Never waste the customers' time with dealership bullshit.

Fourth; have a backbone. If your employer asks you to do something that you know is wrong, make a big stink out in the public lobby and then walk out. Is your time and integrity not valuable as well? I encourage walkouts. I have personally lead 2 of them. It is not comfortable but sometimes it's the only way to prove a point.

On the consumer side, here are a few tips to remember. If you read this last paragraph you will notice they are pretty much in conjunction. First; never buy anything from a salesperson whose face you do not like. Just because they were the first to approach you doesn't make you loyal to them. Ask to see a photograph line up of the sales staff or just tell them that you are searching the lot for a nice salesperson and if you decide that you like them, you will be back. If they are a kind person at heart they will not be hurt by this statement. As a salesperson of many years I would not have been.

Second; walk into the dealership with food. When you sit down at the table to talk, then take out your food and eat it right in front of them. This says two things. That you may be ready to commit to a decision that day and that if they don't give you great service, you are indignant and are prepared to move on without hesitation. If the dealership does not feed its customers then the least they can do is get you out the door in less than one hour with your new car.

Third: ask to see the cost figure for the manufacturer. That is different from the dealer invoice! Then offer to pay no more than say $500 over the invoice price. If they are getting you out the door as quickly as possible then $500 is a lot of money to make free and clear in one hour. Now you don't even have to be that generous but in most cases that would be fair.

We should have a governing authority for used car appraisals. They should be a separate entity from the dealerships. Whatever they say should be what the dealership has to give you if they desire to accept your trade at all.

Still, you should know the value of your vehicle as if it were being sold for scrap metal and know its value in excellent condition. Have a qualified person tell you what your condition is before you even go in. Get that persons qualifications and estimate in writing.

The fact that dealers often credit you more than what they think your trade is worth is irrelevant. This is about them making a sacrifice to earn your business, not about you compromising your position to either get a good trade value or a good price on the new car. Why shouldn't you get both? It's your 6-year savings. Be strong and stand up for what you should believe in, even if you have to walk away from "the deal". There is always another.

As an addendum, I think all dealerships should offer "Just Looking" badges or signs to their customers as they drive on the lot so that they could truly not be hassled. It does happen you know. People do just want to look sometimes.

Can you feel yourself becoming smarter? This is good stuff right here. I for one am impressed with myself.

SPEED & THE DIAMOND LANE

Driving a motorized vehicle is something we take for granted in America. The permit to do so is something that we issue too freely. Obviously we all think that we are the world's greatest drivers, however we can't all be or there would never be any traffic related problems. The first step is admitting that you may not be as skilled as you'd like to be. It doesn't mean that you'll never get there, much as a musician isn't born with the knowledge of how to play the piano for example. It just means you need to practice. The public roads however, are not the place. Hence, we need really large driving schools out in the middle of nowhere. Continue on to page 144.

Is there any American who does not really want to have the Autobahn available for that one time when they really need to get somewhere? Not likely. Even the supremely old and bitter at one time enjoyed the need for speed. True to form - here's the answer. The diamond or carpool lanes should remain only for carpooling as it does promote ecological harmony, but they should be three lanes each, on top of the regular freeways. Speed demons can fly while they mock the rest of civilization. The courageous will test their might on the American superhighways while the fearful (but smart) begin to use the monorail express.

PAYING ATTENTION

Guess what? Green really does mean GO! It means go instantly! Every single car in the line should start moving the instant that the light turns green. Not just go a little either but put the gas pedal to the floor and hold on. If you're in the Pole Position it is your duty to haul ass and waste gas! I'm always ready and waiting. It's the number 2, 3 and 4 cars that usually screw it for the rest of us. One of them is always crouched down picking their nose or something, but they just aren't watching and there is no good excuse for that. If you are the driver you should never take your eyes off the light. Just don't be pussies about driving. Be prepared to give the guy in front of you a little nudge, which brings me to another point. Bumpers need to be a lot more resistant and made completely out of rubber and springs. They should have more than a little give to them because they need to be used a lot more. Come on, we could make those. Give me a break.

When the light does turn green, put that freakin' pedal through the floor every time! Yes, I am repeating myself. Good for you, you're paying attention already. I could be 15th in line and I am ready to go every time. Usually I am waving my arms (or a finger) out the window at somebody. Don't worry about whose behind or on the side of you, and what they think. Don't worry about the cops. Are you worried about getting up to the speed limit too quickly? Unless you jump the gun or have a freakishly fast car and leave smoke and rubber at every light then they are not going to bother you.

I just like to be first. No one beats the P-man off the line. It's that simple. You may have a faster vehicle than I do, but I never loose off the line. Now in writing this I realize that there will be some challengers in the future but you know; that's a good thing because that means the people in the front of the line are paying attention. I don't mind stopping at yellow and red lights because it means that I get to show a few people how a perfect takeoff should be executed every time.

Also, you shouldn't assume that somebody in a big truck won't go off the line fast. Don't try to race someone who doesn't pay for their own gas. Of course you don't know who they are automatically unless the vehicle is stickered. I didn't pay for my gas in a company truck for years and I raced everyone.

ART IN MERGING

Merging is really so simple a thing that everyone needs to be able to do. The problem apparently is that you have to have nerves of steel. Contrary to popular belief, you are not supposed to slow down to look and then proceed with caution. The correct method is to maintain a safe turning speed and then accelerate rapidly to over 55mph. While accelerating one should look for hazards and an open spot. With confidence the driver should then enter the space knowing that it is the responsibility of the person whose bumper is further back than theirs to slow and allow for safe entry.

We could even go so far in the future as to put up lighted signs with laser motion detectors that monitor the traffic and speed, which warn us when it is a bad time to enter or exit a freeway due to low merging possibilities.

Side Note: Never cut off a trucker or other large-scale hauling vehicle. Their capacities for breaking is severely limited and it causes much undo stress and anger. They really do want to kill you when you cut them off, so just be aware of what you are doing. Remember that under my new fighting in public laws they would have the right to take out their anger on you!

LICENSE REVOKATION

My goal is to get the roads wide open. I sincerely believe that we will have to systematically revoke all of the drivers' licenses in the country and re-test the entire nation with the prior knowledge that 70% will fail. This will lead to cleaner streets, less congestion, better air quality, and so forth. This will not go untested by the automakers of course because what would be the point of even trying to sell cars if your marketplace has been wiped out. I am not really concerned about that though, because they are all greedy bitches anyway.

How did Bob Nardelli escape assassination after he fucked Home Depot up the pooper and then who decided it would be a good idea to let him run Chrysler? You know how many people want him dead and nobody is willing to even rough him up a little? I just can't believe that.

DRIVING SCHOOLS

Back to this...upon completion of testing at the new <u>National Academy of Vehicle Skills Enhancement</u> (which again is out in the desert) one will receive wallet cards, rear view mirror hangers, new license plates, and other vehicle insignia and placards which will indicate that you have undergone and successfully passed the most mentally demanding course on Earth and therefore you have attained the full rights and privileges to do whatever you want to on the road; whenever you want to do it. You could even legally and intentionally drive down the wrong side. Not only this but you will be so revered by other drivers that they will get the hell out of your way under the knowledge that if you were to ram their car you would always be in the right. Since you would be an acclaimed professional, they surely must have done something wrong.

Opportunities will be provided for *seemingly* excellent drivers to "test out" as it were in place of actually taking classes. Just like real life college. People who prove that they actually are excellent drivers may be invited to instruct at a very high pay rate.

Initially I or someone equally as cool will have to perform a ride-along with the staff members to ensure that everybody is on the same page as to what will be considered "Acceptable Driving Practices".

I want everyone who is not a licensed professional race car driver to receive the maximum benefit of my knowledge and skill, so here is a potential list of courses at the <u>National Academy of Vehicle Skills Enhancement</u>:

-Hypertension testing and stress reaction timing
-Merging onto the freeway
-Merging onto side streets when you have your own lane
-Exiting the freeway and yielding without stopping
-Completing a turn into the correct lane while in heavy traffic
-Proper signal usage
-Parking Garage Etiquette
-Eating and speaking on phones while in motion
-Taking corners at over 15mph / Shock Durability
-Driving in reverse
-Turning your head to look for obstacles / Mirror Anti-trust
-Green light response time
        (Front, mid-line, and end positions)

AUTO INSURANCE SCAMS

Insurance is the biggest scams in the world. Indeed in the Spanish language, the term "*asegurancia*" is almost like speaking the devils name. It is definitely an American thing. Not all aspects of insurance are bad; necessarily. Deductibles are a crock of shit that need to be outlawed. We pay a lot of money on the principle that if something happens to us or our car that we will be taken care of. That's all. It is not right that we also have to pay even $10 to see the doctor, or the first $250 of the repairs to our front fender. If you elect me president of the United States and subsequently the first elected People's Leader of the World, then I promise to abolish all scams such as insurance deductibles. Oh how the insurance companies like to cry that without deductibles they would be in financial ruin and there would be more fraud, but that is a lie. The term fraud even means "to lie". Insurance fraud is a felony and many people do get locked away for it, so it is not like they don't already police their own industry.

*Insurance agents should not take offense to the previous paragraph as they are only doing their jobs. My father was an agent for 13 long years and made a good living at it, but got no commission from anyone's deductible. Insurance itself is a viable service and a good idea; only the crooked practices should be halted.

Parking is a big scam. We are already paying for the privilege to go see an event. There is nothing glorious about parking that we should have to pay extra for. It's a damn spot of empty pavement that should be free to all people. If we have to pay for parking at least we should have huge spaces that allow for both doors to be wide open at the same time on a full size truck!

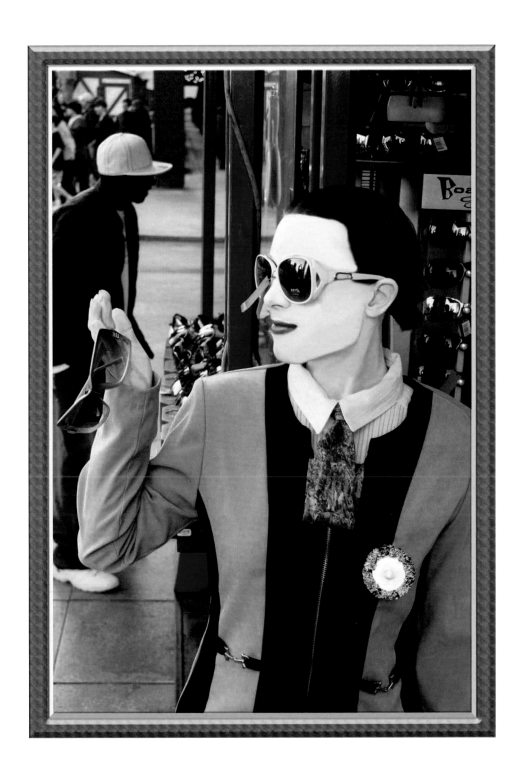

Nipple Suits

These suits are the future symbols of power for the women who command respect and dare to wear them. The user could gracefully cover herself with a scarf to walk into the meetings and for strategic times in her life when she just wants to show a select few. How long would it take for clients to decide to give her the contract or for superior officers to see things her way?

No one could understand the concept of this shot the first time I explained it. I went through several models as well trying to find the right one. Everyone kept saying "But why just the nipple? No one would wear that."

Exactly: "Because no one wears this yet!" until finally after 3 or 4 times they would say "Oh, I get it now". Yeah...the point is to do something different.

This is now officially patented so I expect to be paid by any designer who wants to use one. You bet your sweet cherry ass I'll call you out on the national stage too if you don't. Hey, it's a fantastic idea so let's just have fun and do this thing!

Date Taken:	12/19/2009
Model:	A beautiful, fun loving plaster mannequin
Concept & Photo by:	Parrish Douglas on a Sony a100 10.2mp
Notes:	No external lighting was used. No permissions were asked to show nipples in public. Everyone loved it.

EMPLOYMENT

CHAPTER VII

I am qualified to be the CEO of almost ANY multinational corporation out of the gate - right now. I'm that good.

Just so you know that I am not complaining without rhyme or reason, here is a list of all of the slave factories I have worked at. I call them "slave factories" not because they beat me, but because I felt so uninspired that I may as well have been beaten.

This list is disgusting. From my first job which was picking up trash around the bank my Mother worked for, I then went to a paper route, Taco Bell, Arby's, an unnamed bakery, Schlotzsky's, K-mart, Subway, a mobile DJ company, Incredible Universe, Fry's Electronics, Sears, and about 5 or 6 radio jobs. Cox Communications subcontractor, airport ramp agent, back to Taco Bell for a 2nd round of abuse this time in management, satellite installer, retail display merchandiser and most recently power tool salesman. Intermittently for some temp companies I even did some heavy construction and waste management disposal. That was not pretty. From grunt to manager, I've just about done it all and I can walk into ANY business and give you a large list of most of the things that are wrong in that particular company within 5 minutes.

This is going to be a very complex chapter for some to understand. Again with the communism? Of course all of you will be right in your various respects. I chose to include this topic to eliminate the discussions about what type of person should have what type of job, and why. There is an old saying among persons who commonly debate that reads, "If your point of view isn't ruling the discussion then change the discussion."

I have little doubt that this President can spark the economy into delivering new jobs. It is quality of those jobs that will come into question. Sure we all say that but I mean a plethora of stable, well paying jobs that allow for individual expression and growth. Just keep reading, you'll understand.

I place the economy and employment chapters together because in an idyllic society they are more tightly wound. By this I mean that in the current United States the dollar has no stable value, the rich only become more so and the down trodden have little hope of making it up to even middle class.

OPPORTUNITY

"Anyone can do anything they want to." Provided they are given the opportunity and have the money. "You have to have money to make money." Many people profess to be able to make their own luck, their own fate and their own opportunities. To an extent, one's attitude on the subject can lend one the energy they need to get out of bed and start their journey but if you do not have the tools you cannot do the job and you cannot get a better job.

I guess I'm just pissed off and bitter about the fact that I have had to make all of my own opportunities while some children were given Porches and trips to France. Pretty much if you didn't have to work in fast food, you had an easy life, so bite me.

We hire and fire freely in this country, not according to qualification but more so due to relation, image and ulterior motive. The practice of hiring an untrained worker simply because he's your cousin is totally unethical. Everyone who does so should be publicly shamed. If a child admires their parents role, I say let them study that field in an accredited institution and pay money for that education. Then let them make the same uninspiring journey of sending out 200 resumes while receiving only a handful of rejection letters that state "Wow, we are really impressed by how under-qualified you are yet you demonstrate an incredible amount of enthusiasm. Best of luck to you Sir."

Parents, do your children respect you? Do they mock your decisions then leave the house without regard to punishment? Have they ever put in an honest days work? You can tell a child a story of how you once worked 3½ days straight without food, water, or sleep in the blowing, freezing rain or how you've cooked and slaved over a 400 degree stove for hours but your child will only laugh <u>at</u> you until they can <u>relate</u>.

Let me address your next mental statement. You are probably thinking "The reason we work so hard is so our children don't have to." They will be happy to not have to work but socially speaking they will become "little shits".

If you want them to respect you or learn discipline and ethics then you should do everything in your power to ensure that their first job at the ripe old embarrassing age of 16 is at the greasiest local slop joint you can find. If your child seems to be a popular student, make sure they run the cash register and take out the trash. It won't hinder their self esteem. It might hurt their pride a little. If they are already popular then it is a good test of skill for them to remain so.

If your employer does not absolutely command respect for the superb performance of all their duties, it should be a constitutional right to speak your mind in a public but dignified manner without the fear of being released. I have often thought that maybe a separate institution such as the Better Business Bureau should be set up to oversee such complaints and injustices of the American work force, not however the EEOC.

EEOC

The Equal Employment Opportunity Commission as it stands currently is a joke. The premise is good but the agency does not have the empowerment it needs to really make a difference. There is always a way to get around the current job laws if you really don't want to hire someone. Everyone knows it. Most of us honestly are not given a fair chance at a job we might want and employers know that. Affirmative action is another thing altogether, and I believe we have had a fair amount of progression in that area.

I would like to propose that we adapt a law which states: For every full-time position: An interview must be granted with ALL applicants regardless of qualification -and- before the new selectee is allowed to start, a timely response stating under qualification must be sent to all the candidates.

Finally, since I have a real issue with closure, once a publicly posted position has been filled, every HR Director should be made to issue at least a blanket statement to all applicants stating the name, positive attributes and work history of the winning candidate so that they might know why they were bested for that job and continue to improve upon their own education, skills and training.

This way you eliminate the "waiting to hear" nonsense and a person will know that they had a more honest shot at the job. If a company is found to not follow thru with this procedure, applicants should be allowed by law to throw eggs at the building and defecate on the desk of the CEO.

Thank you, I am a genius.

Now in the support of corporations who really do not want to slosh through the interview process, they should no longer be required to post job openings if they already have a candidate or three in mind. It is a waste of everyone's time and resources. They should however, be forced by law to make an announcement concerning a closed door position filling process. When a person who believes them self to be a qualified applicant becomes shut out of the selection process...they become frustrated. Most of the time a manager has a good idea of who they would like to put in a spot. I say that's ok. Just hire them and let's fix the process so that it is free of the proverbial bullshit.

HUMAN RESOURCES

Most of the people who are in charge of human resources are too busy picking their asses behind closed doors to know when a good candidate even walks through the door. A lot of women seek out this field because it is far more interesting than customer service jobs and it comes with a sense of dominance and power. Furthermore, almost 95% of male human resource agents are only interested in females with little to no skills that they can try to come on to at some point in the future. Same reason: perceived dominance and power. Truth be known; a good HR person who will give a job to a candidate that is clean-cut, hard working and ethical is worth gold.

Continuing on the rampage; what is "Over-qualification" anyway? Let me explain something here, a person can be over-qualified to do many things, but they still need to make a living. End of story.

You need to use this exact phrase when you have to turn down someone who is truly overqualified. "Mr. Douglas, we apologize but we are just too cheap to pay you what you are worth and we are unwilling to make any kind of investment in you since you will more than likely be disgruntled on a daily basis and just leave us anyway." Companies shouldn't hire based on their desire to keep good slaves for life. Too bad for us they do it anyway.

Companies that reward mediocrity by promoting from within make me sick. "Promote from within" is just another excuse to establish a "boy's club" if you will or to take care of somebody's friend who probably doesn't know a damn thing about their present job duties dipping stuff in a deep fryer.

The phrase "REWARDING MEDIOCRITY" © is also mine and is hereby copyright protected. I am not sure that I have the right to even complain about this anymore, because I have certainly become mediocre over the years in my own work ethic. Indeed, I have almost none left.

TO MARKET (*verb*)

Marketing - is marketing, NOT sales! Sales is sales! The term "Marketing" means to <u>promote</u> something or bring it to market where it <u>can be</u> sold. The act of actually selling it to somebody constitutes a different verb. A salespersons job is to <u>sell</u> what <u>has been</u> marketed (past tense). Employers that sell things should not be allowed to use the term "marketing" in their ads. This really pisses me off to no end since I am a "marketer" by trade with skills in the art of promotion, and YOU ARE A FAT BITCH if you think otherwise!

METRICS

My book could never be complete without me telling you how much I fucking hate metrics. God help me if I don't have an aneurism over this one day. I believe I did list this as one of my TS triggers. I think I need a pill and some whisky right now.

If you are a salesperson your boss will inevitably talk to you about how much money you are making for the company and probably some percentage rate of year over year growth. Having been a salesperson I feel qualified to say this: _We don't fucking care!_ No one who is "in the trenches" gives a shit! You know who does care? A corporate VP who's not in the trenches and probably never was. If they had ever been, they would tell their people "I don't care!" I just want to stab my own eyeballs out with the eraser end of a pencil when they start in with this shit.

If you're out there doing your job to the best of your ability and things look good, you'll be fine. If people know who you are and the love what you do then why does it matter? Sales will come, or they won't. You can't magically pull customers out of your ass. We've all tried it. We have national sales conferences where we try it on each other's asses to see if that makes a difference. Conferences just about make me want to rent a hooker and drink all day. Now if you wanted to make customers disappear that's another thing. You could pull a gerbil out of your ass while on the sales floor and I guarantee that would be effective, but pulling customers out really doesn't work.

Could you pay me enough to care? Sure! Fuck yeah you could! Would you do it? Probably not, because the working corporate theory in America is that people on the bottom rung of the ladder shouldn't earn as much. I don't know why that is. They do all the _FUCKING WORK!_

GIVING RAISES

Do you know somebody that works in a dead end job and is barely getting by? Is that person possibly the hardest physically working individual you know? Chances are. Most of the people that have physically demanding jobs, are the most run down of us all and yet they are the least rewarded.

Sure we give raises based on a multitude of things including performance, attitude, cohesiveness, but mostly it's based on if we like the person or not. We find ways to get around fair labor laws. Even though I discussed the minimum $30,000 full time wage in the previous chapter, it is also important to give employees recognition, even if it is to say "Thank you and good job at being a slave".

Merit raises based upon attitude and conformity should be given on top of a raise for attendance and longevity. Give people who have been waiting for acknowledgment the full 25 cents or what-the-hell-ever the maximum raise is. If you are the boss and you put in 70 hours per week, really you still have it better than the grunts.

Fuck it...let's just get of performance reviews all together. I think I am giving up on this subject. 5% every year to every grunt, regardless! Done.

Persons with no personality (i.e. drones) or no moral character should never be promoted. Promote the person who interviews with charisma and has a good idea for change. No one really cares if they have a degree. One of the reasons that I am clinically frustrated and feel the need to write on the behalf of others is that it is increasingly difficult to get a job when you are a sharp person in a world controlled by sloths. How is one supposed to make a living and not go criminally insane? It's not by being faithful to one company for 25 years. I have never been paid enough to be loyal. I get paid to show up. I don't even get paid to look good, I just get paid to show up and sometimes to be a human space heater.

My note to employers and human resource personnel is this: There are plenty of overqualified people out there who can do a job really well for you, perhaps even make you look better. **_They already know they are overqualified_**, but they are making less at their current job and are less productive because they are full of hate toward the system. If they were not willing to accept the amount you are willing to give them, then they would not apply. If you are afraid of looking bad, then you are obligated to tell them, "I am afraid of your potential within this company to overtake my position and I am afraid of change."

Sarcasm wins the race! The crowd is going wild! Yeah... I wonder if a Kentucky Derby horse has ever had that name?

CLEANING HOUSE

Just briefly I would like to say that businesses in general have a power to impact the lives of their employees that just simply goes untapped. All businesses everywhere need to clean house. Get rid of the hose bags. Everybody has one of these people in their workplace and they really know how to make it uncomfortable for you to even go to work in the morning don't they?

Companies have a million ways to get rid of someone they don't want. It's no secret. If you really value your employees, take a survey of the top few people they would like to see go, for whatever reason, and then make it happen. Let the employees vote.

For example: a ballot could read like this...

Employee #2501 Parrish Douglas would like to get rid of,
1. Don Henderson - he's ugly and he smells
2. Carol Wright - backstabber, steals sales, likes gossip
3. Ted Persigal - fuckin' sings country music all day. Metrosexual.

Done. If they get voted off, certainly they should be told why. It's easy, painless and fun for the participants. For the losers - who cares? They are losers! The word "loser" implies losing on many levels to which end you should not care about them. Perhaps if they are smart enough to figure it out, they won't be so annoying on their next jobsite!

THE REVOLVING DOOR EFFECT

This is what I would call the effects of this chapter being put into action. It is the process by which everyone will have jobs that benefit themselves and the community. The grateful community then creates more opportunity and happiness. In essence; one healthy workplace influences another and the cycle continues until everyone feels a little better and then it starts again with the first workplace going to the next happy level.

IMAGINE.

SEXUAL HARASSMENT

There needs to be a clause in the employment laws of this country that says a person has the right to waive their ability to claim sexual harassment and therefore they would welcome most any sexual advances because they are in fact sluts (male or female). I will go ahead and create a rough draft that can be separated from this book and presented to your future employers if you like. See the next page? →

I do this because everyone knows a tease. Everyone works with someone who at one point or another has made gestures or mention of the fact that they would not mind getting it on in a dirty broom closet with you. It's gotten so bad in the last 20 years that now you can't even ask a girl what color her panties are. Come on? Colored panties are fun in a good way and you know it's true. So this form will only help to alleviate any pressures that one might feel about approaching the other party about taking further steps and getting naked on company time!

Do you like nipples sticking out of suit jackets? You're damn straight you do! That is one of my best ideas of all time!

Oh, this definitely called for!

SEXUAL HARASSMENT WAIVER AND DISCLOSURE FORM

I _____, being of sound mind and capable body do hereby forfeit my right to pursue sexual harassment charges against my employer _____, on this the _____ day of _____, _____ and going forward until the time of my termination for work related performance or by my voluntary leave. I understand that this document is a matter of public record and may be viewed by all employees.

By law I am still afforded the right to refuse sexual advances, however only after they have been initially made. This affords all persons the equal opportunity to make comments or to touch my bodily parts at least once. By this document I am acknowledging the fact that it is my nature to be flirtatious and a tease and as of this date I enjoy it. I accept the responsibility that things may go beyond my ability to control a situation, and that I may at times be groped while on duty and on the premises.

Witnessing Company Officer # 1   Date

_____   _____

Witnessing Company Officer # 2

_____   _____

Applicant

_____   _____

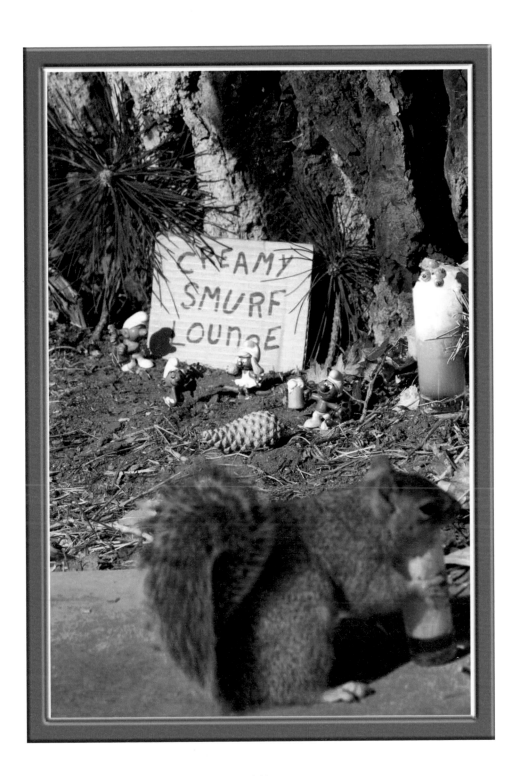

CREAMY SMURF

<u>Public Domain</u>: This is the term I want you to remember. It applies to things that have been created over 25 years ago. It doesn't mean that the Peyo estate doesn't still own the Smurfs™; it just means I don't have to pay them in order to use their likeness for my private use. Besides I did purchase the figurines. You may argue that this is commercial use, but I could have used a Barbie™ and Sound Wave™ as my couple in love, so bite me. The Squirrel did actually come into the shot and boy did he love the cream. It was awesome so I had to go with it. You can't pay for that kind of talent.

Anyway, this photo is not actually about small blue creatures but about relationships in a pure and simple form. I gave my current girlfriend a huge bouquet of flowers when I picked her up before we even had our first date. She loved them. She was a little bit reluctant about being picked up but I requested that she trust me and it all worked out.

Men – don't be lazy.
Women – relax and don't be so mean all the time.

Both sexes – be accepting. For God's sake why be shy? We were created to be together. Start putting it out there and receiving love in return.

Trannies – what <u>exactly</u> is your plan? Bukkake?

RELATIONSHIPS

CHAPTER VIII

***This chapter has had to be re-written several times over and contains devastatingly painful memories for me overlapped with sections spawned from mental anguish!

If I had to sum it all up in one statement it would be this: There are a lot of rules to dating and the biggest one that no one remembers is not to make any rules. Don't be LEGALISTIC. You can't expect to find happiness in your "if/then" little world. It takes the spark and the fun out of everything. Oh yeah, you're guilty. Especially ladies.

Update First, I got brutalized AGAIN _while this was in early editing_ so I had the opportunity to include this little personal snippet. I got destroyed... no better yet _mortally wounded_. My poor old man heart can't take much more of this. It is tough to go through but at least I know that I am alive and living well. I am tired of being devastated because I put it all out there. I might take comfort in that. Then about 6 months later I met a wonderful girl and life is good again. She even supports the release of this; my life's work. I am a person who behaves better when I have a partner. This is time tested. I had been single for years, but I wasn't as nice then.

I have learned, much to my disliking that I smother people with affection and attention. I am going to SMOTHER you and I would very much like to be SMOTHERD in return! Possibly with Knott's Berry Farm Jam. There's no other way to say it. So yeah, I'm often single. Girls run kicking and screaming even though they say I'm the perfect man. It's not my fault. I just want to be loved in return like many of you.

Fortunately, I am told that "creepy" becomes "distinguished" after age 40 and then people just think you are being funny when all along you have never stopped wanting sex with teenage girls.

THE PERFECT DATE

I have several great and hot female friends! They pretty much all confuse me on a daily basis. One in particular has been through 2 pretty rough divorces at a young age, so she has some deep scars and is allowed to feel hurt. I love her dearly but when it comes to the fact that she chooses not be involved with me, I do not understand. I have to constantly remind myself and drudge through rejection and I still can't get it through my head that it's not about me. Relationships are more often than not a tragedy and I'm sure you know someone with a similar profile. I myself had such a lovely divorce that it only bears repeating in person.

Anyway, we had been great friends for 3 years, flirted repeatedly, and admitted that we did in fact love each other, all under the completely platonic roof. She is very spiritually grounded, so we are equally yoked in that way also. I once asked her this question on a whim to figure out why she didn't feel comfortable with the idea of us becoming a couple. *(This is directionally loaded with a right and a wrong answer and I know it's a little out there, but you have to stay within the confides of the scenario)* Here is the very long story question:

"Assume that Jesus returned to Earth as it is now and you just met him. Jesus has his act together. He has no baggage, doesn't need money and is completely happy with himself. For the sake

164

of argument you can assume that he does have whatever it is you think you need a man to have. He has a decent place to live and gets around just fine and he is not going to be sacrificed this time. Assume also that Jesus is the most handsome, generous and caring man you have ever met, so he's perfect! Now Jesus (who knows you very well as a friend since he's God) clearly likes you and has asked you out for a romantic date. What would you say?"...............

The answer _should_ blindly be yes.

You may be thinking right now "Is the author comparing himself to Jesus?" No. Am I damn high on the list of good single men who happen to live in a cave? Yes.

The verses on Love in the Bible that many people quote but few know where it is and fewer still practice loving this way can be found in 1 Corinthians 13: 4-7. Many times it is paraphrased. The key words in there for me have always been "it keeps no record of wrongs". In other words, Love does not keep score. There is no such thing as 3 strikes and you're out. If you live that way and you date with that philosophy, I can guess that you probably have had very little long term success. You are the problem in your bad dating life, get it? Don't do that anymore. First of all it assumes that you are perfect and that's just ridiculous.

CHEATING

I am going to tell you why people cheat and you are not going to like it. When women cheat it always has to do with drugs or alcohol and some bullshit made-up combination of feelings and insecurities. Men are different. Let us start with a basic understanding of Testosterone. It is an inherently evil chemical. Placed in the body of man by God to test us on a recurring basis;

it's basically useless except to Satan who delights in watching men make asses of themselves in public. What I'm saying is that sometimes we do things as a result of high testosterone levels that we know are bad, but the chemical blocks our perception of reality. This directly corresponds to the Sex Chapter sections about masturbation and the big banana.

There's nothing else to tell really. Men don't have ulterior motives as many women choose to believe. We just strongly desire a whole to put it in. Certainly you've seen some mix-matched couples and thought "what are they doing together?" He for damn sure doesn't know! She is just a release for the stupid chemical. It has nothing to do with attraction.

Can you love one person with all your heart and still bang another one? Absolutely you can! I am not saying that I do nor am I saying that it is condonable, but yes it is possible. You women do not get this and I know for a fact you will argue this point to the death. _You think that if we love you then you are supposed to be enough for us._

One woman can NEVER be enough for ANY one man.

Did I just say NEVER? Yes, yes I did. It is called Sin Nature. We are constantly tested by this. It's not about how great of a girl you might be, OK? It has nothing to do with any characteristic you could possibly pick out. It's about vaginas! We like them by nature of who we are! You can't stop us from liking them. You can't hide the vagina because we can sense when it is near like Spiderman™. 99.9% of men need support in order remain faithful. Women absolutely cannot be a part of the support mechanism as it pertains to verbalizing one's sinful desires. If a woman attends a men's meeting, the first thing the whole group wants to do is a gang bang. No women. Get your own support group.

The word "insatiable" comes into play here. One woman is enough for when she is directly touching her man. When you're not with your man his mind wanders. It is an automatic response to being left alone. Simple really; don't analyze it one step further than that. Men don't make commitments to skanks just for sex. That is why we have one night stands with skanks.

Timeless quote; "**Love your man or someone else will.**"

So this brings us to the topic of cheating and how each of the sexes defines it specifically. Since a man is just looking for another whole, is he cheating when he finds one and puts it in? Yes.

Do I think we need to re-define the way we think about sex in relationships? Yes, and my Mom agrees. Sex needs to happen. When you pretend that is doesn't then you create your own problems. When my ex wife left me for a fat slob the issue wasn't sex. It could have been and if it was I was willing to discuss options with her because I did love her. She was inexperienced and young so I could understand if she wanted to try something new. Giving your spouse a list of people you approve of for them to have sex with is not unlike being swingers.

There is hope. Every man will hit a magical point when their bodies will naturally quit trying to hump things. We still want sex but we will be smarter and able to work through the difficulties of not getting laid. You can't put a time frame on it. You also can't force it on us. It will just happen. Just be patient and try to understand. We do love you.

DIMINISHING A CAPACITY FOR LOVE

This comes right after you just learned about cheating for a reason. You incorrectly assume that every human is only capable of loving one other human at any given time. You can love one person for 90% of who they are and a second person for 67% of who they are and still love several other people of the opposite sex for smaller percentages of themselves; but you still might actually feel love for them. It's OK. That is natural.

An integral part of learning to enjoy life is expanding your capacity to love. This may sound ridiculous to many people, especially closed off men, but it should not. It is actually amazing to me that more of our spiritual leaders have not been women. One of the most often heard complaints of women at the end of their relationships is that "I let myself fall in love too fast." They feel emotional stress over this, however it is misguided. They should realize the importance of being able to share their feelings. Returning to the male and the religious sides for a moment; Jesus, Buddha, Dalai Lama, and the Maharishi to name a few all have or had great capacities for love and we are told to pattern our lives after them. Their expressions of love may have been on a higher level than ours, as I do not recall that they "dated".

Why are those who possess and express love after short periods of time ridiculed and not believed? Understanding that love can manifest immediately is difficult to grasp, however don't rule out that something is possible just because you have not experienced it yourself. If you can only relate to short-term love in your past as having been a lie or a manipulation then I feel for you.

When a man tells you that he loves you don't just assume that he is either lying to you or trying to get in your pants or both. Take him at face value and then put him to the test. Show him yourself on your worst day and be moody then see how he feels.

DATING IN GENERAL

Dating is a beast that either becomes your pet, or you fear and hate it for most of your life. There are so many factors involved, not the least of which is the mental strategies that we affix to it. We all think...what-if? The whole thing would be much less stressful if everyone would express what their true intentions and feelings were right from the start. It sounds like a hard thing to do but the pay-off can be tremendous once you have tried it a few times. Back in 1998, I went out with a woman who had an amazingly clear perception of life. After our first date we both agreed that we had a wonderful time. It went at a slow, comfortable pace. At the end of the night before she kissed me she said, "You're a very genuine person." It felt unbelievably good to hear that. I had finally reached a goal that had taken me 27 years of work. We didn't have too many other dates because she didn't want to be with just me which sucked really badly but that's fine and a respectable thing if that's where you're at in life. She couldn't handle it.

There is another side to this honesty thing however. The sad fact is that most of the people you will encounter while being honest will not know how to handle the responses you're giving, and they will run away.

It's very easy to be excited after you've met someone who you really like, and after you've gone out and had a good time. I personally need a shit-pile of attention from my lady. One theory on how to be successful at love is as follows. **Only do 50%.** It's a pretty good theory really. Not mine though and I'll be damned if I could ever follow it. It applies to several aspects of the dating realm. When you try to relate a lifetime of frustration in one evening, almost anyone will feel overwhelmed. I am so guilty of this it is not even funny, but still I continue to try to practice what I am now preaching. Usually when the time comes and I remember the formula it has long since been shot to hell for the night.

Another lovely dating obstacle is what to do when you have no money. This is a real problem since if you really want to see each other there are only about 3 options. The first of these is outdoor activity. You can always go for a walk or hike somewhere. This is unless of course it is winter and you live in one of the nasty winter states. The second option is your old friend television. It's always there although many times nothings on. Your last option does not involve the boob tube but it does involve boobs. It's time to get naked. There are of course several problems with this option. It used to be in the 60's that people could meet each other and sex was accepted and enjoyed as a regular practice. Today people are afraid of being emotionally hurt, getting a disease, or what someone else will think of them. These are certainly valid but can be overcome with honesty and by not dating people who regularly go to places like dance clubs which can lead to hoaring around on a nightly basis. Similarly, you may be poor but that does not mean that you must see someone who is a slob and does not keep themselves or their living space at least decent. This is a big clue to picking a winner.

One final dating tragedy or practice that comes up very often is the giving of advice. This is the one area that entire teams of close personal advisers (including relatives) are more than willing to give you help with. However, before you ruin your partner's day / week or life, look again at your adviser's resume. Is it possible that their lives are 5 times worse than yours? In most cases, yes. This is particularly true for relatives. The last thing they want in the family is someone who doesn't fit their mold. Let's be honest, especially you younger readers. If the parents, siblings, aunts, uncles, cousins, or grandparents find even the smallest thing wrong, your new partner doesn't have much of a chance left with you.

The fact for most of us is that unless you are mentally removed, we care too much about what others will think. What will they say? The gospel truth is that if your family can't respect your judgments or at least act civilized then you don't need them. They may know and even bet money on the fact that you won't last, but they don't have any right to tell you this or to be your judge.

Here's my problem with this, 'cause you know I have some problem with everything. My personal experience was that usually everyone in my partner's family ended up liking me more than my girlfriend did. Here the reverse law seems to apply. "If they like him than he must be bad" and I got dumped. I could never understand what I was doing wrong. I figured that if everyone that she trusted liked me then I was the shoo-in, but no.

The only advice you need for anything in the entire world is this; listen to your heart and soul. They tell you who you are and who you must be. If something makes you happy, then do it. Other strictly good advice would include; being on time. It's a double standard I know but there's no way to fight it if you're co-dependent. You can't be late, but she can. Also, never point that fact out. Women hate to be reminded that they can be wrong. Save your own time by not milling around a noisy, smoky bar room. It just makes you look like a desperate shark. Save that money. Buy one bottle of wine and take it home instead of three or four drinks at the bar each time. Have a nice selection. Then if you ever are fortunate to meet someone genuine you might look like you're prepared and smart. Keep your commitments to your dates if they ask you to go somewhere, but keep your comments (if they're bad) to yourself. When you're out on a date or at a bad party it's ok not to like the surroundings, but bide your tongue and make it up to each other later for the disappointing time you just had.

Personal ads, on a side topic, are something that I have always wanted to try, but never had the courage to. There are too many social suicides waiting to happen, and my time is too valuable to waste on being polite, even for an evening to someone who may have embellished the truth in their ad to the point of a Twilight Zone episode. As a service to the community we need a separate policing entity to review to personal and medical facts for us and to keep ads on the up and up. No more gross misrepresentation of yourself. Ads of the future should read something like this:

Single Male, 29, not messy, no diseases, 27k/yr., above average looks, 170lbs. 25+ previous partners. Likes-going out to eat, classic rock, long sex, sci-fi and action movies. Hates-large social events, driving aimlessly, dogs and cats. Wants-20 to 25 yr. old cute skinny girl who will love me right. I am shallow.

-Or-

Single Female, 43, mild herpes, no income, very attractive, a tall 135lbs. 14 previous partners, Likes-anything expensive, dancing, gossip and shopping, country music, Hates-being hot, bowling/pool halls, sci-fi movies, working. Wants-sugar daddy.

-Or-

Bi-sexual female, 32. Just came into her own. Sexy Bucktooth-Bombshell. Wants an un-confident male, must be less than 4" long/ 1" wide for a fun and loving relationship. I'll share you with my friends! No studs please. I prefer timid and shy men.

So now how does all of this new insight you just got relate to dating more specifically? Men don't see the problems of women strictly as a woman's problems. If we can't seem to move forward with the process of dating, that's the moment when things start to go wrong! We translate any answer that sounds like a "no" automatically into "Damn, well now what am I supposed to do? I can't just turn the switch off." Here are some examples of things that women say and how men perceive the meanings:

"I just need some time for myself" = "I really just don't want to be with YOU right now or ever."

"I have a busy schedule, I'll have to check" = "I really just don't want to be with YOU right now or ever."

"My family is really important to me" = "I really just don't want to be with YOU right now or ever."

I could go on for several more pages, but I think I've made my point. Don't sugar-coat anything. We actually really respect the women who say *"I'm perfectly happy with my boyfriend, thanks but no."* We don't like it when you say that, but we respect it. Here is one acceptable phrase:

"I need to sleep for 3 days" = "Sleep is more important than you."

STRANGERS

Women please, I know the odds are stacked against you, but still all men are not the incarnation of evil. You have some hope, you just need better training on the art of the hunt and you seriously need to take my advice on what men are really thinking. When you ask a man for advice, even if he is completely socially inept, you must trust his judgment more than your own. Especially if you're asking a question about what's on his mind (in reference to your new boyfriend). Trying to think like a man is a lot like trying to think like a computer. Unless you are a trained programmer, you don't have the first clue.

First of all, all men immediately try to picture what you will look like naked. This is unless of course you are a whale and belong in the oceanography institute or your face looks worse than a baboons red ass. Then once he has tried to imagine it, he will then try to see it. Be mindful when you even bend over slightly. They will shift their weight and tilt the head to even see the top 50% of your top. Now there is one thing you can do to alleviate this uncomfortable feeling. Just say right off the bat, "Hey I kind of like you" and open it up and give him a peak. Then just tell him to be nice and wait his turn. I know; it's too radical.

When you hear someone say they want to find somebody who's not "crazy", here's what that means. "I want a girl whose mother doesn't force influence on their lives. They can't make rash decisions that I later have to pay for and they shouldn't have already wrecked their lives (i.e. with children or AIDS infested herpes crabs) therefore they should have great common sense. No offense intended in the previous statement it's just that children shouldn't be having children. I and others like me are not as selfish as you think. We are potentially saving should from suffering on Earth. What is selfish is intentionally getting pregnant because you want a life that will unconditionally love you. That's the pinnacle of selfish. Go buy a damn monkey or a chinchilla.

STRENGTH - FEMINE vs. MASCULINE

My dearest friend Joan and I discussed this topic at length one day. It is the reason that I am not attracted at all to women who put career and money first. Men shouldn't do it either, however it is a masculine quality to be a provider. If she is acting masculine then why would she need me as a man in her life? Makes sense right? A woman can be the president of a company and that doesn't bother me. She can out-earn me by 10:1. I will still desire her if she acts like a woman. I want her to smell pretty, walk demure, hold my hand in public and wait for me. Wearing a full dress in today's society is a completely sexy thing!

LOVE OR LUST

Let it first be understood that this section, while attempting to help differentiate between the feelings of love and lust, is not in any way promoting promiscuity on any basis. I do promote public nudity and voyeurism though. There is no such thing as love until you have been through certain trials. That's just the way it is so don't be upset if you think that you truly love somebody but you haven't been through these yet.

Here are the things you must go through to qualify for being in love with your partner:

1) You must both learn to allow the other to look at members of the opposite sex naked. Either in nudie bars, printed magazines, or in motion video. You must be comfortable in the knowledge that they still want you. It's nothing personal. It's healthy to want to see other people naked.

2) You must never raise your voice to your partner or hang up the phone on them or leave a matter unresolved before the end of the day. No matter what they said or did to anger you, you must never do this or you are not in love.

3) You must learn to trust your partner to go out with their friends of the opposite sex. This is a learned-behavior, and you must do it. Other people are allowed to care about them just not to have sex with them.

4) You must at some point have to put up with your partner when they are drunk or acting a fool. You must baby-sit them and their friends and potentially get up in the middle of the night to drive all the way across town to pick them up. (Personally I recommend only doing this once as a trial because it's really hard to do sometimes, just prove to yourself that you can.)

Once you have mastered these tasks then you have earned the right to say that you are in love and you can then attempt to spend your life with that person. Your best chance for love in this world if you're not already there is to go out with that person you like but you're just not sure of and have fun. Enjoy your life for a change. Go out in public. People who think they have little to no chance of dating you will be pleasantly surprised and will have no inhibitions or shame. They will completely worship you forever. What more could you want? So you might have to mold them a tiny bit over a long period of time with understanding and patience, but it will pay off when you're not divorced after only 3 years.

LETTING THE SPARK DIE

You want to be with someone who's glad to see you. You want to be with someone who verbalizes their love for you 7 or 8 times a day! Attention to your spouse and admiration of them is key. Ladies you also have to work on the affection part over the course of your lives. If the well dries up that is your fault. If the affection wasn't there to begin with and you still got married, then you both have a problem.

Attention and affection are good things, not something to get tired of. If after a certain amount of time you have come to find that kissing your boyfriend or girlfriend does not ignite the same fireworks that it did some time ago, then again you have a problem. Why does it not feel the same way to you any more? How come you're not excited? Chances are fair that you still love that person. If you do love them, the only thing holding back your passion is your own inability to have a good time. Maybe they didn't change, maybe you did. Many of us falsely believe that it is not our own responsibility to keep our relationships fresh, but it is. Where exactly do you think you are going to find this mythical person who doesn't work but has a lot of money, only adores you and spends each moment of his or her day thinking of ways to keep you entertained and happy? It's your fault if you don't allow yourself to still be captivated by your mate, not theirs. Maybe you thought he or she was stunning when you met them, but now you don't. People change very slowly so I doubt that he or she is still the same stunning person you met. They might be doing a different job or have a different car now, but all of that is external. We are all going to get ugly and die. Go find that person you fell in love with again.

When two people meet and decide to come together they go through phases. Although the partners may go through them at different intervals, almost everyone will inevitably go through almost every phase. It is my goal in this section to map these stages out for the world in an easy to understand method. One that a person can look at, identify with and then make a conscious, educated decision to be a part of or to get out of.

1. Acquisition   - Monogamy   2 to 3 wks
2. Probation   - Lots of sex   3 wks to 3 mo

3.	The Hunt	- I can do better	3 to 6 mo
4.	Trial by Fire	- Learning Secrets	6 mo to 1 yr
5.	Commitment	- Living together	1 yr to 2 yrs
6.	End Game	- Popping the ?	2 yrs. on / end

Phase 1.   Acquisition - 2 to 3 weeks

The time at which we decide to stop dating and / or having sex with other people if in fact we ever were. This is the time to tell the other dating prospects that you need some time away from them. Have a few initial dates with the newbie and test the waters to see if they are going to be an exhausting partner. High maintenance is no good.

Phase 2.   Probation - 3 weeks to 3 months

At this mark is where it usually ends for just about everyone at least once in his or her life. It is the natural point at which we have learned about some of the less appealing habits of our partners, we have met some or most of their friends, heard about several escapades, and are forming opinions that will not easily change. The newness is wearing off. We start to become critical and try to fix things that at this point we should leave well enough alone.

This is also the mark at which a miss-match should come to an end. Many people mistakenly think that they are doing something wrong, consistently. They think that they are the problem, when all along they are probably just not analyzing the situation correctly. They are placing more of an importance value on the 3-month encounter than is actually there for both parties. Usually one party will not believe this is the case, but very simply if one person is anywhere close to having doubts, then they should recognize the symptoms, buckle up, be civil to each other and move on. Tons of sex could be getting in the way of you making a good judgment call though.

Phase 3.   The Hunt - 3 to 6 months

This is the time to be decidedly honest with our new partner. If you're going on from here, you have to tell them what it is about them that you don't really like. Maybe they are too hairy in strange places or they dress too sloppily for your tastes most of the time. You do owe it to that person however to express your expectations for them if they would like to stay with you. There are usually more then two things about a person that you won't like and will have to confront them about. This is why this stage is allotted three months. Many times it's hard to find the right time and the right words to say for instance, "Honey I love you, but your breath in the morning smells worse than the dog's ass, and frankly I'd rather kiss the dog's ass, but only in the morning. The rest of the day you're fine sweetheart!"

The other thing that naturally occurs during this time is that you will tell each other (right before the long boring stretch) which of your partners friends you don't like, don't want them hanging out with and why. Sometimes it comes from jealousy, which we have just learned a few pages back that you have to overcome. If the friends in question are indeed "skanks or players", then your partner is the one who will need to concede defeat and let go. Let me just add for a moment that friends will come and go. What a true friend will realize is that you are trying to find happiness and that it is very hard to do. It doesn't mean that you hate that friend or that they should hate your potential spouse for wanting time alone with you. It may mean though, that you won't get to talk to your good friend for a while. That is not being evil, although it can be perceived as such. Take a 1 - 2 year hiatus from your friend and when you come back you'll find that have new things to talk about where it was getting stale. You'll have new insights because someone you love helped you open your eyes, and you'll be testing your intelligence and your ability to handle a situation that used to be uncomfortable for you. You'll be growing. I lost my best friend for 9 years while I was married and then one day we picked up right where we left off and couldn't even remember the disagreement we had.

Phase 4.   Trial by Fire – 6 mo. To 1 year

If you have hidden pornography around your house, then it will be uncovered here, just after your last fight when you thought you had patched every little hole there was. You may be living together now, if only on a trial basis and finding it difficult to routinely clean up after your partner. Guys leave their dishes everywhere. Women leave their cosmetics all over the damn counter. Both sexes leave clothes everywhere, but neither side thinks that theirs looks like clutter. Just the other person's clothes look bad. You of course knew right where your stuff was and you were going right back too it, so it really shouldn't have to be moved.

Phase 5.   Commitment – 1 year to 2 years

Things are good or things are bad. Either way you know by now what to expect for the rest of your time together. You have had some problems and gotten through them, but the real test now begins. You must now decide if you are ready to handle the slow time in your relationship. Some call it boredom. The time when neither one of you can think of something better to do. Your friends may be calling you lame at this point. Long hours at work can leave you too drained at the end of the day to want to go out, but still you feel the need to have something planned, even if it is at home. Personally I am fond of the slow points in life. They define character and they can help you learn things about yourself. Perhaps you're not as interesting a person as you had previously thought. There are a couple of relationship activity suggestions later on in this chapter.

Phase 6.   End Game – 2 yrs. on

Getting Married or Getting Lost. Seriously, after this amount of time (really even one year) you know if you want to be with somebody or not. If you kind of like them but aren't ready for marriage then you need to step up to the plate and say, "I know it's been a great year and I really like you, but I need more excitement." Double date with a new couple and observe how they act. Openly spend time with others and then talk about it later. That will prove to you whether or not you really want them all to yourself. Anyway, if you don't perform your duty and explain that you aren't ready for marriage yet, he will ask you. It's just a matter of time. Most guys who aren't losers don't have a lot of patience for such things. Once their mind is made up that they want to marry you then it's over. They go out and buy a diamond and hope that you won't crush their hearts. You can't tell a guy not to do this either. Just like a Neanderthal: Skull to thick. Can't listen. Big words hurt head.

There are a lot of pretty girls out there that will admit that they've been proposed to 3 or 4 times before and that's what ended that relationship. It wasn't his fault. He was ready to commit. It was her fault for not being honest.

If you have been with someone for many years and they haven't asked you, then just get the hell out. Everyone that you tell about your situation is laughing at you.

There are many people in the world who have simply been scorned too many times. They could love again if they cared too. Not many of these people will ever marry. That's ok. That's their right. We take it upon ourselves to try to cheer people up but if you know such a person; you have a responsibility to be sensitive to their feelings. Here's where it gets tricky. Most of us who know people like this tend to think of them as wet noodles and party wreckers. Although that may be the case, we are the ones at fault for them having a bad time. Odds are that they didn't want to be a part of the festivities at all. How can we expect them to have a good time? In a situation like this we need to learn to walk away. This doesn't mean that you can't still be friends. You just have to learn to say (about a thousand times before it will sink into the skull in question) that anytime they ever feel like going along they are more than welcome.

DECISION MAKING

For many people, making decisions on their own is hard enough. To have to deal with another person's inability to decide is for many of us who don't have a problem with this, unbearable. Nobody likes a wishy-washy person. Those people don't like themselves. Sure, if you are one, you are probably thinking "I like myself fine" and then attaching some profane thought against me for having read into your subconscious nightmare.

Ask yourself, do I really enjoy never expressing myself. Do I enjoy arguing endlessly about where to go until we both starve and then fight about something else? It works on many levels and pertains to every aspect of decisions from what game to play, to which friends to invite, to what time we should set the alarm clock for.

The solution to this undying enigma is quite simple. It starts with the majority of us learning to tell the truth. I myself was a victim of the fibbing bug for many years. When asked by someone else what I wanted to do, the old "I don't know" came rushing out like a pet that hadn't been fed for a week. Then I had a moment of clarity. I now firmly believe;

"Every person, at every moment in their lives, knows exactly what they want." - Me

(That is my trademark caption. Really the whole book is one long quote.) You might want silence and a nap. You might want to get a new boyfriend. You might want to break off a lollipop in your own ass. You might want to dress up in a Toga and watch Revenge of the Nerds on your lunch break. Who cares? It might be stupid, but I am right on this. So never say "I don't know" again. The people who do know, really hate it!

The real problem here is that most of us feel we will be laughed at, scorned, or even deserted for the uttering a bad suggestion. We all feel that. It's natural. If we all feel that though, let's understand and move past it. When the question comes up, say to your partner something like to the following; "I have an idea, tell me what sounds good to you and then we'll make a choice." -or- "I feel like eating Chinese tonight, but if your idea sounds better we can get mine later this week." Don't be afraid of this commitment, your other will respect you more for having been honest.

I have a personal story to relate about and old girlfriend. On our way to dinner, (destination unknown) I asked her what she felt like having. Her reply was so strange that I sat still for a moment to think. She said, "Whatever I decide, you'll just go along with because you love me whether you like it or not." I was so astounded that what I wanted to say couldn't come out. I thought, "What's wrong with that? Isn't that in the job description?" Later I determined that it was her fear of being loved and accepted, along with the new experience of having an opinion that could count for something that perpetuated the answer I received. So I ask you, what's wrong with sharing an opinion with someone you truly love?

LEARNING TO LOVE

Learning to love is a conscience practice, especially if you are in it for the money like my brother Shane. Usually is it not something you would set out to do, again unless you're my brother Shane and you're out to find a somewhat decent girl with lots of family cash. As partners we don't usually walk out the door in the morning and say to ourselves, "I'm going to do some homework about loving today".

When you do find yourself concerned about opening your heart to someone again or even for the first time, here are a few questions you should ask yourself. Remember, don't overanalyze the answers. They are what they are. These questions are designed to make you think in simple terms.

1. Do I trust this person?
2. If I had no distractions in all of life, would I want to be with this person romantically?
3. Are they inherently a good person?
4. Will I suffer any real (not perceived) loss in my life by dating this person? For example: Will I get AIDS?
5. Do they already have a piece of my heart?

If after you answer those you don't have a legitimate reason that you are not open to the possibility of being with that person, then you are either too shallow or too afraid to tell them your true intentions and opinions.

Don't let issues like school or career or distance become confused with your desire to be with someone. Everybody wants to be first in your life before school or work. As for long distance relationships, the only reason those don't work is because people allow themselves to become weak. So one of you has to move, that's not a big fuckin' deal. The person who wants to be with you doesn't have a problem but they own the effect of your problems by default if you can't deal with it.

Once you have learned to accept love, then you also have to accept the fact that your relationship is not going to always be in vacation/honeymoon mode. You have to learn to deal with quirks. I have been sent several e-mails recurrently on this subject. They are for the most part accurate and have to do with classes that we all feel the opposite sex needs to take. You've all seen these I'm sure. A short list included the following:

SEMINARS FOR MEN

COURSE 101: You Too Can Do Housework

COURSE 104: Wonderful Laundry Techniques

COURSE 105: Understanding Responses to Coming Home @ 4am

COURSE 106: Parenting: It Doesn't End With Conception

COURSE 107: Learn To Cook and Fill an Ice Tray

COURSE 205: Putting the Toilet Seat Down

COURSE 206: Overcoming Your Remote Control Dependency

SEMINARS FOR WOMEN

COURSE 113: How to Properly Serve A Beer

COURSE 114: Overcoming Your Shopping Addiction

COURSE 115: Coping With Belches and Farts

COURSE 116: Understanding "Men's Night Out"

COURSE 118: How Not To Be A Bitch When Giving Directions

COURSE 119: How To Overcome "Headaches"

COURSE 310: TV and Big Game Etiquette

Please register immediately as courses for both sexes are in great demand. Class size will be limited to 10 as the courses may prove to be emotional.

Although it was funny, it made me think for a moment. How many people laugh at these but then blow it off as something they don't need to work on? There is humor there that should be appreciated, but then wouldn't the wise thing be to compare the class list to your current and past relationships? If you're not growing and learning, do you have the right to continue to abusively date?

THINGS TO DO TO KEEP IT FRESH

Pick a bouquet of flowers by hand from bushes around the neighborhood. Go for long walks. Hold and kiss her hands. They're very important and centers for stimulation. Take a long drive or motorcycle ride somewhere just to watch the sunset where there's nobody around. Get frisky on the miniature golf course. Take out some paddleboats and try to catch a duck. Always play in public fountains. Make a hideous snowman together and put it on top of your best friend's car hood overnight. Bury somebody's car with snow and wait for the city plow to come along and hit it, thinking its some kids fort. Buy a tandem bike and ride around the city paths. Take lessons together and learn to so something wild or ridiculous. As long as you can have fun together and not be picky about time you'll be ok.

FIGHTING WITH YOUR MATE

I AM right about 90% of the time. When I am not right, I will not open my mouth. That's how I personally maintain such a high percentage. Choose your victories and your defeats strategically. If either party EVER becomes condescending, the relationship is doomed. You can look for all the other warning signs or you can just look for the one really big tack in the road.

Don't ever call someone a liar or use the word lie to their face unless you can back it up with fact and not circumstantial bullshit. Women are terrible about this. People don't always intend to lie; we just don't like to talk about every damn thing that happens to us every day. Sometimes a point that might be considered important just gets left out of the conversation. It's not to intentionally hide things from someone else. Open communication is very difficult to achieve with the people that are close to you and I applaud your efforts if you are a brutally honest person. I know that you have a hard life and I do understand.

Fighting is not really necessary at all if you belong together and you consider yourself to be an intelligent person. First of all, intelligent people are annoyed by the sound of pointless bickering. Also, we hate CNN. What truly drives most of us to argue at all is that fact that we all want to be the person who is right. Isn't that so? Instead of fighting, let me suggest that you instead concede defeat. This serves several purposes. If indeed you are in the right about the topic at hand, then time will prove you to be the victor. Everything happens in time, and everyone who is wrong and likes to run their mouth will always be put in their place, not by you or another person, but by witnessing what you said before being correct and then feeling embarrassed.

In a very basic example; let's say you tell your wife that you took the trash that was sitting outside to the dumpster. When you got home however, a gang of dogs had brought it back to your yard and ripped it apart. If that in fact happened then tell her the truth only one time, then after she calls you a liar (I hate that word) then apologize clean it up and do something nice for her. When the gang dogs return and do the same thing to her, she may not even tell you because she is too embarrassed, but if she does THEN you have the right to cram it down her freakin' throat with a plunger. THEN you can scream and throw things till the cows come home because TIME will have proven YOU to be right.

It's a very strange dance that we do with our partners for no good reason. It is also a very hard thing to trust what your partner says implicitly as the truth. When outrageous things seem to happen to one person more often than they should there is one way to tell if they are habitual liars. Does the story in question get them out of responsibility or labor? If the person has to miss work or is unwilling to claim at least partial responsibility for the incident then they are probably making up some steaming crap. But once in a while, strange things repeatedly happen to nice, good people. It is possible to have a run of really bad luck. If you really love that person though, there is absolutely no reason to get mad and fight about anything.

Allow me to explain something to you. Unless you are rich by a gift of fate then there are only two ways of going through life. You can either find somebody to love with all of your heart or you can be alone. If you choose to love somebody and you give it everything you have then you will be happy. If they leave you, then it wasn't your fault. You did everything possible. Cry for about two days or so then move on. Honestly though if you are really going all out and you are the most romantic and giving person you can be to the point of sometimes exhausting yourself, then there is no way it will fail (unless she becomes a crack whore). The other option in life is to die alone.

Now when I say to die alone, I do not mean when you are old. I mean that if you are not being loved by someone or are in training to live a life of solitude as a monk, then you are dying a slow and painful death. Playing your Nintendo or Sega game system until 3:30 am is a pretty shallow existence if you do it more than once every six months. Am I wrong? Damn, I'm old.

So don't fight with your mate. It's not worth it. Don't fight about things that don't matter like who does more housework or how often. Housework is just something that we do to occasionally do to pass the time. You shouldn't get mad at your other because they are typing on the computer while you are vacuuming the floor. If they are engaged in something that is important to them or they are working on a resume for example, then they are attempting to make life better for the both of you. It takes time though and people are exhausted after work. Sometimes you need to do something by yourself on your day off. Not for the whole day, but let them have an hour or two ok?

BREAKING IT OFF

Every single relationship in my entire life has ended for some really stupid-ass reason. Oh yeah, I'm qualified to write about this.

If it's really just time to go, then don't beat around the bush. There are definite signs that point toward the end of the road like when she doesn't want to hold and swing your hand in public anymore. Lack of affection in public is like the ax coming down on the chicken's head. That's the one true sign that it's over. When the time has come to end your relationship, ABOVE ALL ELSE, be honest and take responsibility. It's really simple. If you decide that you can't live with someone who has bad hair, then tell them. If their face looks like it got hit by a truck but they are a really nice person, you owe it them to say it straight. <u>Somebody has to be the bad guy</u>. If it's you, then you have to suck it up, admit to yourself and the other person that quite frankly, you're too shallow to continue a relationship with someone who's not absolutely perfect.

By doing this you accomplish three very important goals.
1. You have just alleviated yourself of any guilt.
2. You at least win respect points for having been honest.
3. The other person, having learned of their horrid traits, can now use that knowledge to better themselves and can continue on with future relationships having felt the obvious closure.

Understand this also; most people feel the need to break up for one of two reasons; because you're on the crazy train -or- you didn't want to be a couple in the first place but you got stuck.

Never say this, EVER → "It's not you, I promise." This means: "A lot of little things about you bother me and I am really SUPER shallow. I can't tell you what those things are. I am also weak minded and I act like a child, plus I am afraid you'll punch me in the face for being stupid, which I am."

Also never say this: → "I didn't mean to hurt you." So don't then! If you really want to make amends we're going to have to have sex at least 5 more times while we talk about this.

This last comment completely needs to be addressed and is actually directed at the ladies because no straight man would ever say this in his lifetime. "I think we need to cool down because it seems like you just want me for sex." Woman … hell yeah it seems like I want a lot of sex because we just started having sex and I like it! We need to have a lot more sex before we can slow down and build something. We are in the sex phase! Of course it's going to seem like I want you for sex because I do.

That doesn't mean I don't love you. You just have to wait it out. It's natural! The Sex and the Building Friendship phases do not go together. They barely overlap.   It's only ever OK to talk about not having sex if it is a matter of your religious belief.

REVENGE

"Living well is life's best revenge." Mafia Joe. He also happens to be a cop, but not dirty. He does the deeds for free. After my divorce we were talking about recovery methods. It is absolutely true. If you just can't do it that way though I am all about old fashioned revenge and giving it to people that hurt you.

Start with something offensive and ride it all the way into the morning. For example; shave off all your pubic hair and put it in a nice little box. Send it to your ex with a note that says, "I won't be needing this anymore so I thought I would send it to you as a memento. It just gets in the way now and frankly we're usually too covered in sauce to deal with it."   Even if this really isn't the case, the fact that you did that will really fuck their perceptions of the entire world.

If they really burned you bad, then make it a point to contact them whenever anything really good happens in your life. Send them postcards from Italy. Send pictures of yourself with several naked people and flowing drinks for all, drive around their neighborhood block 6 times in a limousine full of screaming friends. Have people call on a regular basis and ask for you. Little annoyances to let your ex know that you are better then they are. Sometimes that's what it's all about.

LEARNING TO FALL

I have a dear friend named Erin that I completely fell in love with in less than a day. She mostly hides from me because I am a bit overwhelming. I get that. We were in Spain at the time and I am pretty much a hopeless romantic. She was in a relationship at the time so we jointly respected the boundaries of that. The feelings were mutual though. She told me something that I didn't expect to hear. *"I think it's better to love even if it's only for a short time."* I already felt that way but she confirmed it for me. Moments of love like that will stick in my mind for a long time.

When someone tells you that they love you, take that at face value and assume it is true. It might not be your definition of love and it might be a little clouded. Be accepting and gracious. If you feel the same way, then express it! What I do want you to do is talk about it later; say the very next day. Give it a little while to sink in and for you both to feel comfortable. Then it's the perfect time to establish what you both think that means. You will always have expectations of someone once that is out on the table. By openly talking about it you're not allowing them to fail.

Pure honesty is something that 99.9% of the population will never achieve, but it is a goal that 100% of the population should have. Although many of us feel it is wrong to express our true feelings about another person, the reluctance of doing so can be very damaging. Suppressing such feeling can blow out an "O" ring and damage a liver or burst a spleen or something. Don't hold it in. It's not healthy.

Remember all the things you just read in this chapter and start being nicer to each other. Start giving more and taking less. Don't make a sacrifice to be with someone you don't think you can love, but don't make excuses when it could be right there in front of you. Trust your gut feelings, even when you're scared.

Do I still believe in true love you ask? Do I believe anything can be forever? I do believe in love at first sight, you just have to let yourself go, but remember you do still have to go through all the same steps. Just because you fell in love quickly doesn't mean you get a hall pass through the hard times. I do believe that love can last a lifetime. So far for me it has, but for the women I have loved it hasn't. I respectfully reserve the right to say yes that it did happen until the day I am on my death bed. It is sad. I truly, truly hope it does not take that long.

THE SECRET
OF THE PLOT

I Love You...A Lot

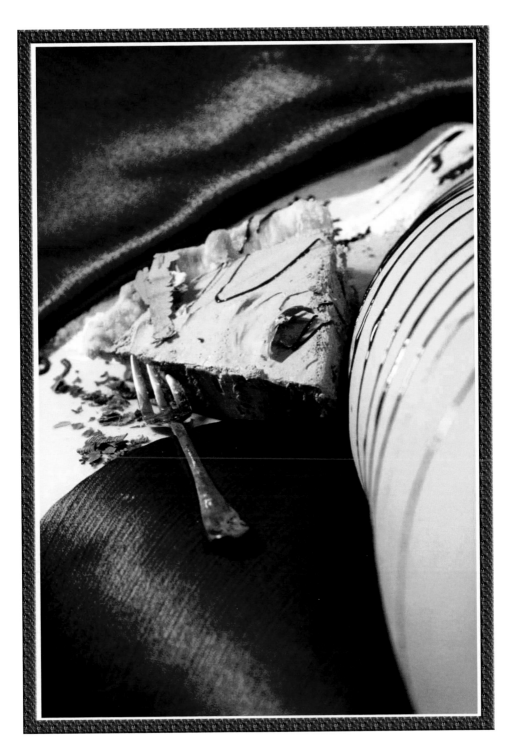

"FRENCH SILK PIE"

It is of course one of the most appetizing and sinful deserts that one can imagine. My mother's kitchen produces one of the best. The slice of delicacy is placed here over the woman on what we refer to in America as "the pie". To add the more basic element for understanding, a silk sash is draped over her body as well. The woman in this picture was selected to have a creamy white or milky skin texture that we often times associate the French with having. To be correct, it is not to say that they are pale, but rather that they are fair in this rich and desirable state. Although a fair skinned person is not always immediately desirable to every type of personality, the image here serves "literally" to represent that there is beauty in everything and that sometimes we are foolish to look beyond our most basic elements.

Date Taken: September 2009

Model: I can only say she is closely related to another model in this book. Completely awesome girl to whom I owe a deep debt. I refused for years to publish without this particular shot.

Location: My Home Studio

Concept By: Parrish Douglas

Photo Taken By: Parrish Douglas

Pie Made By: Mama Sharon

SEX

CHAPTER IX

Now it occurred to me that I was half way finished writing this book and I had selected most of the photo shots that I wanted to go between the chapters, but I had not even started a chapter on sex yet, so here it is.

Let's start with this; Tiger Woods is a lying douche bag. He's not addicted to sex more than any other man on the planet. He just got caught and therefore has to make up an excuse. I am addicted to sex and so is every other man. Thank you.

Moving on; there are a whole lot of people in this world that really don't know the first thing about sex, and for all we like to talk about it on television and radio, we are still skirting the issue. People want to know how to get it done, how to get it in there, and how to make it good for both parties. I promise you that if you read this chapter in its entirety that you will no longer be in the dark my friends. Sex is awesome. Sex is wonderful. Sex can be downright funny. (Insert "queef")

In my school we were taught that God created men and women differently so that we could join in sex and thereby glorify Him. I buy that. It makes sense when you think about saying "oh God" during the middle of it. In religious context we are supposed to be married.   The interesting thing about being divorced and having a sin nature is that it is awfully hard to revert to celibacy.

Sex is a lot of things, but it should never be used as a tool and it should always be taken seriously. That is a little preachy I know, but the premise of using it to gain something is entirely evil. Sex can cause a damn lot of problems. Right at this very moment I am sitting in a mall, editing this book on my laptop and watching little 14 year old skanks running around. I am just embarrassed for them. Actually I'm embarrassed for all the skanks and I am in the clean, upscale suburbs today.

SEX FOR HETERO'S

When you look at something like a woman's body or a flower or a landscape or a building in a city, look at it as though it turns you on. I do this with pancakes. Look at it through the perspective of a high definition lens that allows you to see the minutest details at every angle that you wish to view. Look at your husband or wife this way.   You will see how beautiful they are.   Life is exuberant that way. It puts you in the correct frame of mind for being with someone special.

Now to start off with, sex is better with noises. Most everything is better with noises, but mainly food and sex. Don't be afraid to make them because you are actually telling the other person that you enjoy what they're doing. Most people are too embarrassed to make noises, but shouldn't they be more embarrassed about showing their naked ugly bodies to someone? I think so.

Ladies, you can add a lot of unnecessary stress to a new sexual situation and not even be aware of it. The man is really doing most of the work. I would like to say otherwise but there are few women out there who really like to move and know what they're doing during sex. Not being aware of his potential "Performance Anxiety" can add exhaustion and frustration on top of the nervousness he may already have. Give him a break ladies. Offer to play with him first or even to try the 69 position. It's very relaxing and it gives him the chance to play without feeling guilty. Most of all it's important to remember to have fun and to never be visibly disappointed. The world is not full of sexual studs that can just ride all night long.

From the man's perspective, it is sometimes entertaining to place just a little bit of distance between your two bodies so that he can see what is going on. That's the reason people buy porno isn't it? To watch what happens? So it's natural to want to watch when it's right there in front of you. As far as motion is concerned, guys generally like to move it in and out the entire length of their penis. It just feels better. Sure it does make them ejaculate much faster, but that's what it's all about. Feeling good and losing the load. The most damaging thing you can do to your sexual relationship is to stop having sex immediately after he releases for the first time. If you encourage him to continue, it will get better over time. As a general rule, men who regularly engage in cardio-vascular exercise will have better stamina in bed. This will of course depend on both how long it has been since he had sex and if it is the first time for that day.

Men also like to release and to see how far it can fly. It's just a manly thing. Don't try to understand. More on understanding these compulsory actions in a few pages.

You have to take turns and share. For the woman it feels better sometimes to do something completely different. If you really want to please her then you have to learn to behave and give sometimes as well as receive. What you are giving is the favor of allowing her to have it her way and that means more than you realize. *This little section is written with the help of women so don't think that I just made it up.*

Women like to feel close to you. They have made the choice to be with you and they would like some consolation of the fact that you want to be close to them as well. Sex with distance between your bodies is just too impersonal for many women and that's fine. You have to be sensitive to what she wants first and then if you play nice for a while she will open up to you. Women like to feel you inside them with a slow motion. Speed is not as important as being together. Unless you are both agreed on having a fling, you will probably not last long as a boyfriend if you play too rough.

5 QUESTIONS

I thought it would be fun to do my own little independent study to find out (and publish to assist you the reader) what the top 5 sexual questions that one gender would ask the other would be. Now the questions are different for a good reason. When you try to find a few average males with only average sex drives, you discover that such a person is not average and is very hard to find. The average male is a sexual deviant and therefore the questions that an average male would ask a nice, average, unimposing, non-hooker-like female are always going to be deviant.

By contrast, the average female (although they do have some of the same desires) would not normally ask such explicit questions due to their reserved nature. Now I am talking about the average female and here is where the difference lies. Not every single woman is a deviant. Almost every single male is, and they're open about it as well. So the questions I received are as follows. You may or may not be surprised. What I think you should do with this knowledge is the next time you are out on a date volunteer your answers to the five that pertain to you and take the night from there. You might really be surprised what you can accomplish once you are open about it.

The Top 5 Sexual Questions Men Want To Ask Women:

1. Would you ever have three-way sex with me and another girl, and do you know any other girls?
2. Do you like to give head and will you swallow?
3. Would you ever lick another girl's pussy?
4. Will you have sex with me in weird places?
5. Would you ever try anal sex?

The Top 5 Sexual Questions Women Want To Ask Men:

1. Are you willing to experiment with toys?
2. Do you like to have the lights on or off?
3. Have you ever had or wanted to try anal sex?
4. Are you willing to get tested for diseases?
5. Do you like to be gentle or rough?

Other noteworthy questions included: "Does the fat on my body really matter?" and "Do you even really like me?"

UTERUSES

It is also noteworthy to mention that in my independent survey, it was found that women who have had a hysterectomy did not generally care. They tend to feel like they have already had every type of sexual experience in the world that they cared to have and for the most part they were unimpressed. I cannot in good conscience say that they are totally right or wrong but they most definitely are in a different category than women with uteruses, and therefore it might be wise to take sexual advice from them with a grain of salt. They can usually tell some great stories about the sex they had when they were "with uterus" but if you ask them what they would currently like to do with a physically studly man, the answer can range from depressing all the way to "Why would I even care about that?"

MANANAS

The penis truly holds many mysteries for many women. To understand it you must first learn that it is really nothing more than one giant oversized exposed nerve. It's a nerve ladies, trust me, I have one and it is quite large. Being that it is a nerve it is connected to other muscles and causes reaction in them when activated. It magically points the way to moist things; including but not limited to cakes and pies.

When you accidentally hit the tender spot on the inside of your elbow called the funny bone it sends a wave of pain and mysterious pleasure through your entire arm, in like manner when your pheromones even come close to a sensitive penis you are in effect sending pleasure and likely some future pain through the man's entire body. The pain will probably be more emotional than anything else. Now like any machine, it has one main control option. The penis has one switch. It is the power button. Actually it is more appropriate to say that it is always "on", but there are certain stimuli that can act as a circuit breaker. Big ol' fat people would be one such instance for me personally.

When trying to get the machine to work it is always good to remember that "wetter is better". If you would like to use some kind of lubricant in place of bodily fluid it won't know the difference, but you'll have less trouble with that sucker if it's lubed up. The body tells us that it likes lubrication by inadvertently giving us nocturnal emissions when we are young. Sometimes these can be quite funny and scary in retrospect.

Fortunately I still have the extremely sexual dreams; however I have foregone the "wet" part of them. Now that I am older though, I actually achieve penetration in my dreams whereas young boys do not. That bit of knowledge is solely intended for you women, and really I just wanted to use the phrase *nocturnal emissions* in a sentence because I find it wildly amusing.

Let's explore the sections of the penis and what feels good to which parts. First you have to include the little guys; the family jewels. If I haven't mentioned it before, it is always a good idea to get these cleaned up by method of shaving. No one likes a hairy mess. Just shave them down; it doesn't decrease your manliness. In all likelihood your female friend will appreciate the fact that you considered her feelings about your anatomy. You respected her enough to not look like an ape.

One really should not try to play with the jewels too much by hand. They are not receptive to this. They only respond to a gentle tongue and only for the first five minutes or so. Once they get used to the initial shock of being touched then the stimulus response decreases quickly. It is only the initial shock value that sends waves of pleasure through the body. In reality that feeling is equally as comparable to that of ejaculation and so it is not a bad idea at all to do this to your mate early in foreplay to rile him up and make him more receptive.

Now the base of the penis, when large or small, only serves to hold the thing on. Holding it by the base or starting your stroking method from way back there really does no good at all. Only the underside where the tube is raised is even remotely sensitive. Just forget about grabbing it there until you are experienced.

There are two parts to the mid-section. Under close observation you will notice that a circumcised penis has a ring around it where the skin changes from tan to a sort of pink. This is actually the mark at about which a man can no longer "hold back the tide" so to speak. This mark should also be the center of your hand stroke. The said stroke should begin with your hand just below that mark and continue up until just after touching the ridge at the top section. This will maximize your response time. Pulling up any further is completely unnecessary and it hurts if he has ever had a hernia operation.

Finally the tip of the penis isn't actually all that responsive either. Only the underside off the ridge is receptive. That is the target always and forever. Only during actual intercourse does the full stroke count, but for different reasons. At that point men instinctively think that giving their partner a full stroke makes the sex better. Whether or not it actually does depends on the female but the man will then to think it's all about him.

BREASTS

According to a T-shirt that we bought for my brother Shane when we were in Honolulu there are 15 major types of breasts. These are bee stings, pointers, blockbusters, has-beens, pears, bananas, head lights, peaches, cucumbers, double bubbles, watermelons, cantaloupes, flap jacks, gum drops, and coat hooks. I am partial to peaches, pears and pointers myself. I guess you would have to see it to laugh as hard as I did but you get the mental picture.

Boobies are a very nice thing to have and I am actually quite jealous that I do not have them. If I did have them I would use them to my fullest advantage and try to get as far in life as I possibly could without actually being slutty. Those are some powerful things those boobies. Damn near magnetic. If you are a single, remotely good-looking girl you owe it to the world to show those things off. Not just to anybody and I'm not suggesting that every girl should be a nudie bar dancer. Certainly not. I am merely saying that if a boy is being nice to you and acting courteous, if you think that he is cute you should give him a little peak that's all. Good boys deserve to see more nipples as a reward for being good. This goes for your neighbors as well. If they are good neighbors and help you out then showing your boobs is just a way to say thank you, much like a handshake. Thank you.

HAVING AN ORGASM

I can't for the life of me figure out why girls claim to have them so rarely. Just let it go. Squirt all over the fucker. Ladies, it is your body. By all means you should know when something is feeling good to you. So why do so many women hold themselves back from having an orgasm? It's not like you're making a gigantic mess like us men. It doesn't mean that you are going to shrink and then sex will be over. Just let it happen and _make plenty of noise_ when it does. If you're not going in with the intention of getting something out of it then why bother? That's all I have to say. I have several female friends who say they have great control over their timing and you should too. If you don't then get together with some of your friends, work it out, try different things and then talk about it later.

THE MAGIC WOO-WOO

Allow me to first get into how to care for the vagina while in a sexual situation and then I will cover some other less appetizing points. Being the soft and warm apparatus that it is, it should be cared for delicately. You've got to kiss and lick that thing sometimes for a good hour so that she feels cared for. Now you've got to look up once in a while and make sure that she's not getting bored. You can't just "paint the fence". Sometimes you've got to get your tongue in between her lips and then apply a mild squeezing pressure from both sides with your fingers. Sometimes you've just got to attack one side of it and the lack of balance will drive her crazy until you've hit the other side, but it keeps the interest focused on the act and on your presence.

During the act of intercourse remember this; it's not about what size the man is, it's about how often he hits the contact points. Ladies, you know where they are so for your own sake help him out a bit if he doesn't get it. How is he supposed to know where they are if you haven't told him! It's not in an exact universal location for every single woman! If he isn't hitting the mark (or even if he is) try throwing one of his legs over yours but keep the other one on the inside. Now don't let him put distance between your bodies, as his tendency will be to do. Keep him close and just move what has to be moved. You're not wasting energy and it will keep him going longer.

"Ah, Master Parrish, so there are a few secrets" you say? "Yes children," I reply. "It is both a science and an art. You have much yet to learn."

It helps quite a bit to use this general rule in developing your own techniques: If it would feel good to you if you were a girl; then do it. Obviously if you are just with someone for the first time or for one night, which happens...nobody get mad here, then you don't want to take the liberty of showing her your freaky twisted side. If you have a freaky twisted side then you may want to at least bring it up at dinner on the second date, purely out of respect.

Ok, now for the descriptive stuff. When a ladies genital area is left unchecked and becomes hairy, men affectionately referred to it as "Napalm". The first time I heard my two brothers coin this in a sentence I almost urinated down my own leg, mainly because they are both younger than me. In like manner we have dubbed the finely shaven vertical single line to be "The Landing Strip".

The clitoris is up near the top for those who don't know. It is usually receded a bit and hidden under some folds of skin, so you can't expect to be hitting it if you're not changing positions once in a while. The best description I have for it would be like a clear pink marble, about one quarter the size of a standard pearl. You would have to be looking with a fair amount of light to actually see it, and until you know what you are after you can't expect to feel it either. Ask a good friend to play show and tell with you. Make sure that you are nice and tell her you could use the help and would appreciate the favor.

Flaps or wings as they are sometimes called are a fact of life, but the correct knowledge about the flaps can help you to make the right decisions about your potential partners. They *can be* (**not necessarily are, but likely to be**) clear indicators or windows into the past at certain stages of a woman's life. For instance, when you run across flaps on a young girl, let's say for legal reasons she's 18. The human body is supposed to be fairly resilient at this point and the lips should return to their normal states of pillow-like being. If they do not and she is 18, this is a clear indicator that she is involved with a lot of drinking, possibly drugs, is either a whore or easily taken advantage of, and she is lying to you when she says that your only #5. The truth is that you are #50, but she cannot really be expected to tell you that at her age.

Remember this, "If it's brown, turn it down", unless she is of Latin-American decent. That's rude you say! Yes, yes it is. Go ahead and argue the point though.

When big-ol' flaps are encountered on a woman who is recently divorced, you may assume that she had a good sex life when she was married and that that probably was not the problem. You would be foolish at this point to try the "lots of hard loving'" angle. If you do, just be advised that she will leave you soon as well. This woman is probably in her very late 20's to early 40's and needs emotional tending and a lot of vacation. On the other hand, if in this divorcee she has retained her pillows then I guarantee there is a hidden issue. One of the two of them had a problem and you at least have half a chance at being "the man".

Now if you are married and you and your wife don't have that much sex, but one day you notice that over the course of two weeks or so she has converted from pillows to flaps, then you may have a problem. You feel me here?

POSITIONS

There are some positions that are outright just hard to master. For instance, standing up in the shower takes a lot of balance and can wear you out easily as you may not be used to standing like that. The water can also cause problems because the additional pulsations of the water on his skin may lead to sensory distractions and shrink the man. It may also delude the woman's natural lubrication. You women out there have got to be more sensitive about being dry. Sometimes it is your fault if he can't get it in there and in all my field research I have yet to encounter one single woman who admits to being dry. Damn it all!

From time to time people have difficulty with the rear entry position. I have two names for it. The collision of pelvis to backside creates a sort of butt-wave that a surfer could ride in. That's what I now call it, "riding the wave". I use it as a term of endearment really. Since there apparently is no clinical term for this position I have created a more scientific / reference style name for it as well. (Yes, I did go to the library and look for a while) It just seems wrong to me that you would have to use the term "doggie" when you are trying to hold an intelligent conversation so let's call it the *Rodillum Position*, referring to the knees in Latin based languages. Right-o-then. Carry on.

Anyway, trouble you might experience in this position could be mostly due to a simple height difference, wherein you either have a man with tall legs or there is a lot of distance between the woman's vagina and her rectum. Some women just aren't centrally located. It's just how they developed and it is nobody's fault. It can even make sex in the standard missionary style difficult. Some girls have the thing almost exposed out in front while others have it back with not even a half-inch between their two openings. We usually call this the "Taint" or the "Gooch". It's a darn shame that sometimes two people just don't fit sometimes, but what are you gonna do?

Don't give up on experimentation. Whichever of you is the male; try lying down and putting one leg up in the air, or sit in a chair while she gets on top facing forward. Put a leg up on the kitchen counter or let her do a handstand with her legs apart while you lower yourself down from a bar mounted on the ceiling. Sure it takes a little bit of strength and doesn't last long, but you could say that you did it! One more thing, and this one's for the ladies; men ALWAYS want to try having sex in the movie theater and on airplanes. Just try it will you?

THE MISSIONARY STORY

This story comes to you from my close friend Vivian. I'm sure it has a foundation in the truth but it is her unique choices of words that make the story really come to life and have new meaning for the reader. "It seems as though when the early American settlers were expanding their way across the territory they came into contact with various Indian tribes. In an attempt to bring them to Christianity from their crude religions, missionaries of the church were dispatched to spend time with the Indians and to help them understand and bring them to be civilized. When it came to sex, the missionaries found that all of the Indians were doing it

209

"Doggy Style", and this was savage and unacceptable. So they taught them the correct way to have sex with the lady lying down and the man on top, and thus it became known as the Missionary position."

MY EXPERIENCE HAS BEEN...

Every single person who has had sex has done it with someone they shouldn't have. If you don't take the safety whale out once then you don't know what good really is. You don't appreciate it. If you treat your partner like royalty all of the time, you never tell them no and you give them your unconditional support in every instance, they will have to make love to you all the time. Get it in your contract. This is much the same manner in which I seduced your Mom but maybe you've blocked that out by now. I had her face buried in a pillow and she was screaming due to the nature of my largeness and perfect rhythm.

Yeah that was uncalled for. I was definitely writing loaded when I was sitting in Earnest Hemmingway's front lawn in Key West, Florida with my drawers on my head. I am relatively sure that was also uncalled for...maybe.

Now then; I have had some very good sexual experiences in my life. Occasionally when I am with a new partner there is the random incident of limpness, but this quickly passes once I settle myself down and realize that I am just with another person who just happens to be a goddess. Perhaps a better term would be stage fright. I have to commend the girls this has happened to for not leaving. But as an old friend of mine used to say when we were drunk and in college, "It all comes out in the wash". I remain confident that my lovin' was the best they will ever encounter in their lives. That's how I force myself to go on. I pretty much embellish, but then again I am a writer and as such I have certain liberties.

Here is an excellent life lesson that is definitely true. Ladies; "love your man or somebody else will." By love I mean fuck, OK? It is in man's nature to crave sex. The sin of adultery has already been committed in our minds. Don't give your man the opportunity to stray by just allowing yourself to believe that you should be enough. You're not sweetheart and you were never meant to be. It's all about how intelligent you are. The best thing to do is to keep him tired from humping you all the time. You also have to at least talk about the kink and have a future plan for it. If you just like one kind of sex then you better like being a bachelorette.

AFTER PLAY

This is a new concept for a lot of people out there, but it works just the same way as foreplay does. It eases tension and smoothes the transition to the next part of your day or night. Continue to arouse each other after one or both of you has reached climax. Don't just go to sleep. Kiss each other some more. Get back into that 69 position. It's very fun and you shouldn't have to be worried about what it's going to taste like. That is a damn stupid question that you have created in your own mind. If you have already committed to letting the other person have sex with your body then you might as well finish it the right way. Going to sleep immediately after, even though you are holding each other, is not necessarily the healthiest way to finish your encounter on a regular basis. You could try massage. Everybody likes that right. Maybe write I Love You notes on your partner's body with a pen. That will last until tomorrow.

HORMONES

Perhaps I should put this under the Theories chapter but it is just as well that it goes here. I believe that we could solve a large number of the world's problems if we took out the hormones in our youth. I'm talking about developing a means to hold back the development of things such as breasts until the age of 19 and then let them start to grow. Likewise, a counter-agent for testosterone should be developed. Not estrogen but something else that won't turn little boys into sissies, but will just diminish their lustful desires.

If we held these things back until such time as our young became adults and had better reasoning capabilities then they would be a lot less likely to commit crimes against women and the rest of society. We could hold them to more accountable standards for their actions if they did. We all become enraged when a 14-year-old kid commits a major felony and then is only sent to rehab or juvenile detention for 3 months. This way we could punish the little bastards the way we should be able to.

This would reduce the rates of date rape, assault, vandalism, shootings, theft, and whatever else you can think of. (Actually estrogen might be a good thing for kids in old gang neighborhoods and for prisoners too. That's another brilliant capital punishment idea.) Now in answer to the people who will say, "That's all fine and good but we wouldn't have any great memories without things like sex and booze and breaking things and stealing. We'd just be losers and geeks." Well I say you're pretty much losers and geeks now so what's the problem? You just dress a *little-tiny* bit better.

Most kids don't know when to quit. They burn themselves out on violent habits and really aren't that productive later in life. If we set good habits for them at a young age they will be great loving adults who truly know how to appreciate life. By the way...we don't even have real ghettos in the United States. If you think you are impoverished, go live in Nicaragua, Haiti or Africa. Go get AIDS and not be able to afford oatmeal to eat or to rub on your wounds.

WHAT LITTLE GIRLS ARE MADE OF

Now that I have told you about controlling hormones, I can freely admit that I like young women and I fully intend to surround myself with them for as long as possible or until I die. My ex-wife, I am happy to say was much younger than me. It is not to say that younger women are any more attractive than women in their 30's or 40's, it's just that usually they don't enter a relationship with all of the preconceived notions that most women past 25 have formulated. Men are probably the same way and so I do not blame anyone who engages in robbing the proverbial cradle on either side. I like them young but one cannot have the fruit from the vine until it has aged for 18 years, which is still certainly acceptable of course. So until my theories of hormone reduction can be enacted, IF you don't want persons with less self control than I have groping and licking your daughters THEN you shouldn't be havin'em!

Post Script: It is cool to be a virgin for all of you young ladies out there, even for many years and well into your twenties or thirties. Every young woman has a special luster, which is lost forever upon having sex for the first time. The only one who can see it is the man who proclaimed his love for you and who shared that moment with you. Choose the man you want to share this with carefully. It is better to go with a nerdy, less attractive guy (if you must lose it) that will pine for you for years to come rather than someone who is just out for bragging rights.

This is just a reminder that a real man can respect innocence, and appreciate its beauty, even though he will want you all the more. The moment he realizes you have had sex with another man, he will no longer lay down his life for you. That is an awfully large amount of power to lose. I have said it before, if I were a woman, I would rule the world.

So it is then that being in a virgin state is a powerful thing for a woman. Even the image of a virgin in a magazine is powerful and it can compel a product to sell better. This is why we often see pictures of young women in "school girl outfits", with the pure white shirt and the little plaid uniform skirt that just covers her perfect round bottom. Damn that image. Private schools really need to consider a dress code change to baggy, unattractive slacks with square padding.

So as not to get too far off track and to finish the chapter, a real man can also smell a skunk from ten miles away in just the same way that we can all see a drunk from far away, so don't be too much of a slut unless you've decided to make it a profession. It looks bad and people love to talk. If you're going to be a slut, everyone will know before you have the chance to let on. We can tell it in the way that you walk and stand and by the way you roll your eyes at the cashiers in the grocery lines so you might as well act the part and get naked in public all the time.

Don't be a tease. That is just plain annoying. Just start flashing people, get naked, work it girl, be that slut! Yeah!

(At this point if I were planning to stay in the U.S., I might get some therapy. This is a seemingly long chapter and I have embarrassed myself at least twice...)

MASTURBATION

Making butter, that was always a good one. Waxing the dolphin was popular in my era also. Whatever you want to call it there has to be at least a hundred euphemisms for it. Performing the action whether you are a male or a female is not wrong and it does not make you a bad person. In fact it makes you healthier, and admission of the deed can make you a stronger person. Science has proven several times over that the release of the body's natural sexual frustrations leads to a more healthy and productive mind. Thinking constantly of sex forces us to revert to a more primitive state of being. The longer we think only about having sex, the more primitive we become.

So who else is going to do it for you? Who else is going to touch you in the way you want to be touched. If you have somebody that you can trust enough to talk to about what you really like then that's great, but even a lot of married couples don't enjoy that freedom. I don't have a lot to say on the subject except that as you get old you really don't care so much anymore. Old meaning 32-ish.

GAYNESS

If something is labeled gay or IS gay in neon colors, then it is obviously bad! That's the end of the story right there! The word "gay" doesn't carry with it the sexual connotation for me at all. It simply means that I am vehemently opposed to something, so first and foremost you should be on board with that.

I have to write about this because everyone inevitably asks me my opinion, so at least by writing it down I won't have to repeat myself as much.

As far as whether or not I believe it is wrong, yeah I do. I just think that you people think it is something different to do for a while at a certain time in your life. You must be viewing it as experimentation. I will come back to this point again but I believe that God really does care about you being straight. More importantly though God also cares about you being a good person to the rest of humanity, so if that's what it takes...fine. There are bigger social issues to fix that outrank gayness. God allows us figure things out for ourselves. If you choose to lick the crotch of a same-sexed being, I think that might set you back a little when trying to gain entrance into the proverbial heaven. Not a lot, but maybe a little. Way more so if you are a man. Judges?

Now I only know a few gay women. Their choice does not bother me at all. They are great people because they have discovered what makes them happy and that is their partner. Once you have a good partner you can then become a better person by not having to devote so much time to looking and acting.

Also, women are the more attractive sex. This is fact. They are called fair because they are pleasurable. Their parts don't have big disgusting veins sticking out and they generally don't smell as bad as us. The girls that I know don't prance unless they are world class dancers. I would of course like to know every hot lesbian and be invited to watch but that's probably not going to happen. I might be a lesbian if I was a woman. Definitely bi-sexual.

The thing about lesbianism -v- homosexuality that many people don't understand (this is a glittering generality) is that lesbians (prior to this book) do not understand men very well. Homosexual men do understand women though. This has nothing to do with riding dirt bikes or wearing different hair styles and clothes.

I understand that it's about finding someone who is capable of loving you and your sofa king retarded self. We all have issues; some people find it easier and more comforting to be with someone of the same sex who can better relate without all the hassles. A much greater percentage of lesbian and gay people are very happy in their relationships and most heterosexual people are really not.

So far as gay men are concerned, prancing around is totally unacceptable anywhere in the world. If you prance and someone does happen to call you a "Faggot" well you pretty much earned that. I don't use that word at all. I have mentally trained myself not to. "Fucking homo" is the default phrase that comes out of my mouth and I find that I use it to describe predominantly straight people that I still don't approve of :) It's awesome.

What is also awesome is what a great job they did with the movie _I Now Pronounce You Chuck and Larry_. Great messages, great writing and its totally believable that people act in that cruel of a manner. I do not condone cruelty towards the gay community.

You as a reader are not authorized to put words in my mouth.

I don't hate them. I just hate prancing and high voices. That's all. Honestly, I don't tolerate gay people very well when they prance around. It's a trigger for me. I immediately desire to mame and destroy gay men. The fact that they floss their teeth with the flagellum of another man's sperm does bother me yes, however not so much as the ridiculous way they act. Yeah, I said flagellum.

I just don't understand the need to prance around limp-wristed, wear embarrassing clothing and speaking in a tone that is not their natural voice. WHAT'S WITH THE FUCKING VOICE CHANGE, REALLY? I just don't get it. I have met quite a lot of gay men in my life and 98% of them like to dance around and throw themselves at everybody just for attention.

That's where gay people get a bad rap from and that's why they sometimes get roughed up. "Heretos" cannot tolerate shit like prancing for very long. It is like a screaming child right in your ear. Just don't do it in public and there won't be any problems.

When you speak to a service representative in any field (ESPECIALLY TRAVEL) just use your normal voice and stop being a damned fool for two seconds. Then you can go back to having your fun later. The person you are interacting with doesn't want to be at work anyway so don't make them listen to your queer spewing vocal semen. Cock pigs.

Just one side note; I have always thought that the airline industry should support a "Queen of the Runway Pageant". That would be fun for them and funny for me. I would watch that, although it would have to be in segments so I could stomach it and not die laughing.

So I don't care what you do in your off time. I am not the keeper in Purgatory and besides the gay population equates to less people in my dating pool. There are too many people in the world for that to be an important concern of mine. I am pissed off about enough things in life. Furthermore; *THERE IS NO GAY GENE!!!! YOU WEREN'T BORN WITH IT!!!! YOU ARE A FUCKING LOSER!!!!* Why do you think you have the right to make up this bull-shit gay gene? Where **_EXACTLY_** does gay fall on the double spiral DNA helix or is it on the molecular chart after Iron but next to the phosphates? I forget. Go spend all the Gay money in the entire world on research and find the gay gene (not the hetero money from people who don't care). Show me the gay gene and I will gladly print a retraction. I think that is fair.

If my child told me they were gay, you bet your sweet ass I would punch them right in the face and then duct tape them to a tree in the back yard so they could have some quiet time with the universe to figure things out.

There is a cure to gayness. It's called punching! Sometimes it takes a few doses. Like 200 maybe. The shit that television promotes. Really...

Now this is the most simple and yet wonderful question of all. I love it. I never get tired of it. So here we go. "What does the Bible say?" The #1 best-selling book of all time (like it or not) the Bible...reads as follows:

LEVITICUS 20:13

*"If a man lies with another man...both of them have done
what is detestable; they must be put to death.
Their blood will be on their own heads."*

OK, so that's pretty bad yeah? This is coming right from God through the mouth of Moses. I'm not trying to put anyone to death here, but clearly: gay = bad. The blood reference means that if you are prancing around and some random hetero goes into a berserker rage and attacks you with a beer bottle you may possibly have brought that upon yourself.

Also, just so you know, the next few verses go on to say don't be having sex with farm animals. I know some of you like that stuff. Mexicans guys when I worked at the airport have actually told me that they put it in chickens to prove their dominance. That's fucked up but true! Clearly we are living in different times now and there are more women than pigmy goats, so guys your odds are better with the real chicks. I do believe that God loves you regardless of what you choose to do, but clearly He didn't intend for square pegs to go into oblong shape holes if you know what I mean. I am pretty damn sure you do.

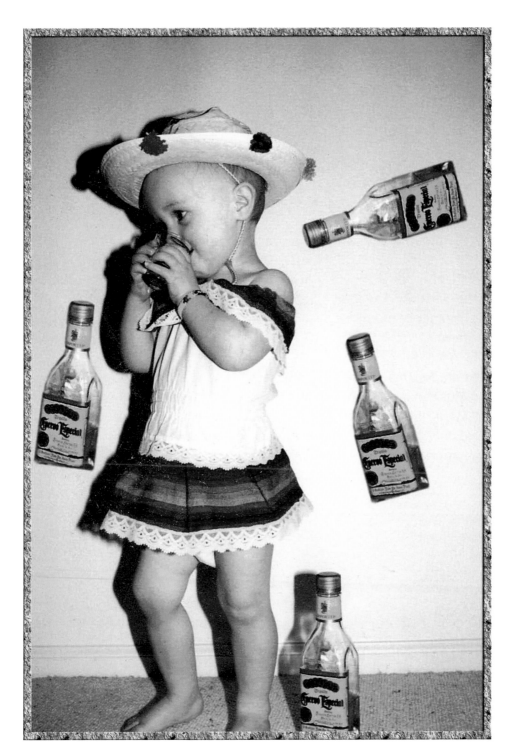

"Cubanos Blancos"

So the point is...parents should be allowed to make their children drink so they can have a break. I thought I would drive that home with the extra bottles. The one on the ground is of course the original. Get an expert to examine it. I promise it's real.

For those of you, who think you have the right to comment on my photography skills, fuck off! This happened in real life and real life also has shadows. I just captured the moment. Yes the child is wearing a diaper. So again I say, go fuck yourself with a cheaper brand of tequila. Heradura brand maybe, extra gasoline flavor.

I am also aware that the title says "Cuban" and yet the girl is in a Mexican dress. My family is messed up. We act like Cubans. My Cuban friend Vivian gave us the title so we can use it. We just didn't have any Cuban dresses at the time ok? I love all nationalities and I do speak Spanish very well so don't hate me, cool?

Date Taken: Summer 1998

Location: a hut south of the border

Model: My niece Kara

Concept-babysitting: Parrish Douglas

Photo Taken By: Parrish Douglas

REPRODUCTION & CHILD REARING

CHAPTER X

Children are basically Ugnaughts™ made for slavery at Bespin.

Ugnaughts™ that should in no damn way have any technology like fucking I-pods™ until 17 years old. We didn't even have shit like pagers until about '94 so I want to know who was the first pussy-ass parent who gave in and let their kids have cool stuff. That's why our kids are losers. They don't get out and do stuff like play.

Damn this chapter seems long to me! I am definitely going to catch *more* hell for this chapter than for any other. I expect it from every one of my friends and family too. Just remember, I am not saying I don't love your kids. I am not insulting children here. My intention is to directly insult the adults.

Look around you. As you do so, keep an open mind to things such as diversity, which make our culture rich. Do not focus on clothing or hair color (even if it's green) but rather on disease, poverty, obesity, starvation, etc. **We all must take a hard look at ourselves and decide if were truly ready to have a child**. If not, there are options. I will propose some that you have probably not even thought of before. They are certainly not the only right ones, but I think you'll be inclined to agree that they may help a great deal.

Before you read on you should also understand that some wonderful children have come from otherwise disturbing persons and disastrous relationships. These are strong individuals at this point in their pre-teen lives, which have had to sacrifice a lot of things just so that they could survive virtually on their own and still learn how to function in society. Maybe they are even still holding strong into their teens, but how many of them will survive in the future without developing the same types of problems and disorders themselves. Personal growth and development does not stop when you reach 18. Adults develop bad habits at the same rate as kids do, but we are afforded the luxury of being able to do things at strange hours and behind our own closed doors where many of them cannot. Parents simply believe their kids are being deviant because they have to sneak around.

I have plenty of close friends that have had children at a very early age. To my limited knowledge they are good kids and I am glad to know them. I don't necessarily think that the time was right for their parents to have kids though and I think their lives would be much different now had that circumstance have been delayed. For some people, having children defines their being. Without a clear direction in their lives it becomes something to do to fall back on. It's a way out. The expectations to do something grandiose with their life have been alleviated because they are now a parent. That should not be a reason to have a child. It is not amusing that it comes down to selfishness a high percentage of the time.

GOD'S ROLE

Many will undoubtedly argue, "It is my God given right to do whatever I want to with my body!" Please be civil and continue reading before you may be inclined to make a public display.

Conventional thinking may prematurely lead us to believe that this chapter is going to be anti -or- pro-abortion. I assure you that it is neither. Like every other chapter, it is pro self-control.

God has a miniscule role in procreation. God simply supplies the soul. We do the rest; so don't blame God when something goes wrong. If you have a child out of wedlock that does not mean it was your destiny. It means you were stupid for one moment in time and you had bad judgment. When you stick it in unprotected, what do think is going to happen? I'm not an unrelatable asshole. I've pulled out and prayed before; and yes I was a stupid jack-ass. That's ok. Let's grow together.

We all wish that there was a sperm/egg compatibility time frame of say 2 months. Imagine men if your sperm were an away team from Star Trek. You send them on a mission; they find the egg and report back to you by radio. If things don't look good -or- if the captain makes a bad decision in the heat of the moment because he wanted to put it in the green alien woman, then you could just transport your whole sperm team back to the ship with no harm done. That would be awesome! Unfortunately for us, things are not that way.

Now on the other hand if both you and your spouse have been fixed (cut, tied and soldered) and you still have a baby, after you get the blood work back that proves you two broken people are the parents, then you can claim destiny and Immaculate Conception. That's fair.

It is a fact that 90% of the people living on Earth today believe that there is a God. We worship in many different ways. We pray for a lot of different things. Have you ever heard the prayers of a child who is being beaten by an alcoholic parent, or one whose parents fight all the time and as a result they are not allowed to play like a child should. Some of them pray for their parents, but some of them pray to be taken away or even to die. That shouldn't have to happen!

You as an individual bear the _ability_ but not the _right_ to procreate. Every time you choose to exercise that ability, you are playing God for a moment. You are the one who is condemning your child to a life of servitude, working in a retail store or fast food place. You are the one who is deciding that a being should be created and be made to go through the ridicule that comes at school if your child is not perfect in every way. You are the judge that has decided that your new little life must even go to school and sit through what many, many kids consider to be torture. (If you are smart enough, patient and dedicated, I see nothing wrong with home schooling.) If you have a fat kid or a weak little runt or a butt-face ugly child with braces from here to eternity, you did that to them! Just remember that you owe them whatever retribution they demand for the rest of their lives.

Their little free spirit that you pulled down from heaven or wherever to inhabit the body of your child; they were a perfectly happy soul in a life of bliss, possibly having already gone through life before. They didn't ask for the pathetic life you may be giving them and God doesn't want them to have a pathetic life either. God wants for all of God's children to be happy and prosperous. Sometimes, we just make it happen the other way. The reason is because we are **SELFISH** or **GREEDY** and don't consider the life of children to be as important as our own when we choose to have them. You flat out owe it to the soul that will inhabit your baby to consider all of these things. Personally, I am very pissed off about being made to work and I think that your baby will be too.

226

THE GOVERNMENTS ROLE

I am a firm advocate for government regulation of this process. If couples cannot meet the humane requirements set forth in this book to protect the lives of their children from un-necessary hardships than I believe that the government should be allowed to step in and take custody of the child, relocating it to a better suited home. Forget about love for a while. <u>Love can absolutely be bought</u>. Not all the time and it is not for sale to everyone, but yes it can happen. As long as the home is warm, there is good food, lots of quality attention and the child gets to pick the toys they'll be able to put off memories of their old life until they are grown enough to revisit their real parents and show them what a shining example of humanity they have become. They may even choose to tell their old parents off, which would be their right if they chose to do so.

Once under the governments' control the child will have a very secure and well cared for life. It may not be the happiest time for them but some wonderful things could come as a result from such a program. Once having hit the appropriate middle school age, individual leadership skills can grow. Children could be groomed at an early age for success in a given position. Success makes everyone happy, and there would be a relative assurance that it would actually happen. All the while the children of the government are being taught the knowledge and skills they will need to perform in life, they are also being responsible, respectable and well mannered under threat of military control.

Only if a child is a serious misbehaver should we then use them to conduct experiments or send them away for special training. No win scenarios, kamikaze pilots and missions to Jupiter, things like that. Of course that stage of the game is a bit cruel but you as a parent were a loser in the first place, so they did not really have a chance. You gave them the loser gene and it is hard to overcome. At a certain point in time the child would have proven to be a loser too. You can call me an evil tyrant, that's fine. You won't however, be able to say I didn't warn you to be a better parent before they come to take your baby away. You might become a better parent for the fear of that happening.

PERMITS

Taking logic one step further now, I firmly believe that people should be required to get a reproduction permit from the International Consortium of Human Evolution or something of the like. Apparently the idea of this has been touched upon before in several mediums. I thought this must be another unique idea of mine until I saw the movie Starship Troopers in which was made reference to a regulated control of birthing rights. Obviously then if it was incorporated into a science fiction movie then at least someone else must think it's a valid idea. Ideology and the enactment thereof is how society changes and grows for the better. You must accept this. Many of the things that I make mention to in this book will come to pass. I may be dead by then and not able to say that I was right, but time will prove me right.

The initiation of a permit system does not however mean that we will be outlawing sex. That would be ridiculous unless we did not have the sufficient anatomy and only mutants had working parts or something like that. Sex is too important for our survival. It feels too good and helps our minds to function from day to day. Have all the sex you can handle, just don't reproduce.

Requirements for a reproduction permit should include.

- Both parents to have no criminal background at all, including juvenile crimes past the age of 14.
- Must not be more than 40 pounds overweight.

- Must have had stable employment in any field; or regular employment within a field of expertise totaling 4 years.
- Monetarily, a combined income of three times that of the established national poverty level for a couple.
- Both parents must belong to a church or viable civic group of some kind; either of which must outreach and help its community.
- Both parents must be at least 26 years of age.
- Both parents must be fully self-aware. (If you don't know exactly what this means then you're not even close. Sorry, try again.)

The reasons for some of these guidelines should be self-evident. I would really hope so.

ADOPTION

I have decided to put the section about adoption first, lest I be stoned or flogged in the streets. I've seen rallies.

Adoption is a wonderfully viable solution to the desire to have a child. It is hard to go wrong with this option from either viewpoint. There are thousands of qualified parents every year that try desperately to adopt. The rules are very tough on people who are trying to get a child as well. You do have to prove your worth so to speak. The people who chose to adopt are great human beings, and they *usually* raise exceptional children who come to have good lives.

As far as giving it up goes, that is far too hard a thing to do. I admire the courage that it takes to let go that these women posses. I cannot even imagine having the strength to do such a thing. I have chosen not to have children myself by having a bionic penis, but I would very much like to adopt someday and raise a child. I would love the opportunity to give someone else a wonderful chance at life, but only when I am ready.

I really cannot write about this subject anymore because I find it an emotionally hard topic for me. I only choose to include it because when you run for a position of power in the world, which I at some point would like to do, then everyone inevitably wants to know your position on a few subjects.

ABORTION

Allow me the literary liberty to begin with a little comedy. Sperm isn't smart enough to seek out your intelligent egg. Sperm oozes down your uterus until it accidentally finds a well placed egg. Want proof? Go pull some sperm from the factory and put it on the wall then see what happens. It's not going to swim up the wall even if there's a perfect egg one millimeter away from it. Thank you!

Personally I don't believe abortion is such a bad thing. No I don't believe that it's a human yet and I don't believe that it has a soul at conception. The fetus does have human characteristics, yes. If it already had a soul it would be really, really bored for 9 months and maybe go crazy. Technically it doesn't fall under my criterion for even being alive until the heart beats and it shows brain function by movement of muscle groups. I think the laws governing abortion are just fine the way they are. Maybe they are even a bit loose. Really, you should be smart enough to know what you are doing by the time you very first start to show. I would say that anything past 4 months might be pushing the envelope, but who am I to say? If a mother can't decide by that time, well then she would first be an idiot and thereby fall victim to the rules of the previous segments.

Let it be known that I do feel bad for unborn babies. If you stick a picture of one in front of me I will probably get a little weak.

Separately, jokes about abortion in the 70th trimester are damn funny!

Really I don't have that much more to say about the subject. I do think it's a viable option for many women in bad situations. I do think that the "Morning After" pill should be made readily available and over-the-counter in the United States. Accessibility is the key for many young women who wouldn't otherwise know where to turn. If you can't give the child everything that you wanted when you were a kid, then you owe it to at least 3 people involved to consider the option.

I do have one thing to say though about being a single mother. Now of course I know nothing about being one myself, but I would like to offer a perspective. Something for potential mothers or girls to think about if they were to be considering keeping their children.

In this paragraph I am asking you girls to be selfish for just one minute. Think about all of the other things you want in your lifetime besides a baby. Do you ever hope to secure a good job? Do you still like to date around and flirt with men? Would you like to eventually get a nicer vehicle with a good stereo that you can use to take vacations to other states or maybe to Mexico? Of course there are anti-discrimination laws in place to make sure that you are afforded the opportunity to still get a good job, but they don't honestly count for much. Your world will change and you will only be treated in the same manner as people see you. Unfortunately, men control a large percentage of the private sector and many men view a single mother or even a young mother as a problem waiting to happen. Why should they take a chance on you when you have already proven yourself to be irresponsible in their eyes? You don't think you are irresponsible, but what you think doesn't really matter anymore in the big world. One would also assume that you would still like to find a nice guy.

Here's a hint. Nice guys are usually very smart guys and they never want baggage. There are a very limited number of nice guys out there that will tolerate taking on someone else's child. I am one of those guys, but it has to be the right mother and the right child. You might as well invest heavily in the lottery as to try to find one on your own. Even if you do, they still would prefer you not to have any. A child is not something that you can go back and erase, and it will not go away for a long time. If you became pregnant in a bad, unloving or irresponsible situation and you ever hope to change your living conditions then you need to consider some option and you only have two to choose from. Just remember, studly guys with green eyes and the cash to match don't want you. Can you honestly say that you think the best thing for your life is to continue with having your child?

CLONING

This is some scary shit folks. To think that science has developed the way to breed people from vials to be mostly the way we want them to be. This shit is real too. It may come to pass in your lifetime that a human clone causes some chaos in the world. When I die I want to stay dead and be remembered as a legend, not as a thing that just keeps going and never changing.

I don't even want anyone to clone one of my organs to keep me alive a bit longer. I say if my original shit breaks then too bad for me. Life has a course and a lot of the time life can be filled with a lot of superfluous nonsense that we don't really need or want to deal with. Do you want to be cloned so that you can continue to work your fingers to the bone 5 or 6 days a week? "Not I", said the brown cow. If you have the life of a millionaire playboy and you've had that level of comfort all of your life, then maybe.

RESPONSIBILITY

There are entirely too many people in the world. It's that simple. The basic gene pool has been split way too many times. How can everybody even hope to be playing with a full deck? A full deck contains 52 cards. When you shuffle your deck with someone else's, you are trying to cram 104 cards together and then chose the best 52 for your child. What is most often happening though is that some of the good cards fall on the floor and are lost, while still others who make the cut have greasy potato chip stains on them and still others are ripped and bent. Because it is in our nature to be lazy, we don't raise ourselves (by that I mean our standards) to get a new and still smooth deck. We just accept the damaged one and thereby condemn ourselves and inevitably the next player to losing. Understand?

If you are fat and stupid then you will probably need someone to translate the fact that if you are fat and stupid and you reproduce with someone who is fat and stupid, then your children WILL BE fatter and more stupid than thou, and the circle will not be broken. The moral of the story here children is "Always wash your hands before you get into bed with your cousin." What?

Unless my destiny brings me to be extremely wealthy **AND** married to a wonderful, beautiful woman, there is no way I would have considered bringing a child into the world. In fact that is my gift to mother earth. To have one less wretched soul, sucking on her teats and draining her of life for 80+ years.

CHILDREN IN PUBLIC

There are fewer joys greater than watching ones child laugh and play without a care in the world. There are few annoyances worse than watching an adult child trying to control a real child. Part of being a good parent is having and utilizing the knowledge that everything you do must revolve around the harmonious evolution of your child. As much of a crime as it may be to have to pay a lot of money to do things with your family, it is a crime more so to punish a tired child and a tired community by forcing the pursuit of fun. We must "learn" to set our expectations lower in terms of what we can accomplish when with children.

I use the term "learn" very strongly. Typically we do not take naps every day as we did when we were little. Ask yourself; why not? We must remember and then re-learn that down time is an essential element to a healthy spirit. It is known that many people who faithfully meditate live well beyond their expected years and rarely have health or mental problems.

METHODOLOGY IN PROBLEMS

You may feel free to use any and all of the following methods on anyone where the situation merits, regardless of age. I realize that this may have serious workplace implications for some of you, and that is fine. Anyone who is acting like an infant should respond to the same stimulus.

For the purpose of protecting my friends from media inundation, I will use alias names for them. These names by the way I do think are fairly cool and if I was to have children I would at least try to give them these names. I am told they would be swiftly voted down but at least they are names that would give a child room to grow. Take for example the name Zues. The girls could call him "Z" and it would be a cute thing, but for him it could create pride and give him a domineering persona. For a girl I have always like names like Cassiopeia. She could be Cass or Cassy to her friends but the longer version is powerful and sexy and she could use that to her advantage. I sidetracked there...back now to the problems.

Method #1; It's all in the Presentation

I tell this story to all of my friends that have children. I assure you that it is 100% true and witness verifiable. One day in about mid 1993, my good friend Bob came to Omaha from a small town about an hour away with his three girls (then ages 4, 3, and infant).

While at a stop at my parents' house, the two older girls were playing next to the kitchen where my mother was completely engrossed in a cooking project.

Soon the older girls erupted into a fight about who was playing with a particular dolly. They both had dollies, but one had left hers in the car. Before their father Bob could even get out of his chair, my mother used her magic and reached into the cupboard pulling out a regular, unopened 5-pound bag of sugar. She then said, "Girls, look over here! I have the best thing in the whole wide world! I think it's even better than Dolly!" Both girls responded with just electric excitement, "What is it, what is it?!" After a skillful pause, "It's SUGAR!" my mom said, "now who wants it?" "I do, I do, I do!" and then the debate became about who was the better behaved girl and deserved it more. We could only watch and learn from the master.

At this point Dolly could have been recycled for all anyone cared. It stayed that way. Mom told them about all the cool things sugar could do and about all the things that you could create with it. She had all the conviction and energy of a television preacher. They were powerless to move.

She later came over to us and all she said was, "It's all in the presentation." Bob was powerless to respond and I was still laughing.

Method #2; Revocation of objects

This story involves several instances over an extended period of time. It was necessary to use time as a teacher here in proving to the parent that their method of dispute settlement perhaps needed a tune up.

The several instances took place everywhere you can imagine. In the car, at McDonalds, at home, at the movies, at the grocery store, etc... The children of Robert would fight over the ownership rights to everything. As a friend, an onlooker and a child of master parents it occurred to me that there was a better way to handle such a problem. I remember suggesting several times that he and the girls' mother should try taking everything away and telling the kids that the adults owned everything and that they were only being nice in letting the kids have use of it for a while. Not wanting to be wrong, they continued to do things the way they saw fit.

One day the opportunity arose for me to play the shepherd. The family of Bob was staying for the night at my house because they didn't want to make the long drive back home to the country. The girls were given their own room, but were loud enough to get our attention in another part of the house. When I went in to check on them with father close behind, they were waging war based on who should have the red pillow and the yellow blanket with the stripes. Bob finally agreed to observe this time and allowed me to take all the sleeping paraphernalia away and leave them cold and on the floor, claiming that everything was mine (*which this time it was*). If they just wanted to fight, that would be ok, but I was taking all the prizes for myself. Within five minutes, the peace treaty was signed and all the nations were observing a blackout.

This theory can and I think should apply to everything in the home with the very, minutely small exceptions that should absolutely only be made with Christmas and Birthday presents. Children have as great a capacity to learn both good and bad habits as adults do. If they learn not to be so ridiculously greedy at a young age, that's one less thing we all have to complain about when they grow up.

Method #3; "Cry for me!" My Fathers Angle

My father had a wonderful take on crying that I learned to appreciate and use when my younger brother Shane came to be the crying age. Now this was not used recklessly. If the situation warranted and Shane were hurt or had another legitimate complaint than the proper attention and care were paid. On the contrary, if the crying came because someone was looking at him, or breathing on him, or if we touched him at all then this is what he got. My Dad would very lovingly pick him up, look directly at him, and in a gentle understanding (but secretly mocking) voice say, "cry for me baby Shane. Come on, give Daddy a big cry. Let EVERYONE see how good baby Shane can cry." Another amazing magic trick! Don't even think for a second that a child can't interpret the feeling of ridicule and decent. Performed in the loving facade though, it proved to be the perfect medicine.

As a side note, my other brother and I did repeatedly pick on Shane and I in particular liked to squeeze his lingering baby flab. In hindsight this probably had some scarring effect.

Time outs: The Losers Way Out

I think that what the term "time out" is saying to the child is "go away"; I don't want to deal with you right now. Time out only indicates that you are frustrated and the child has beaten you down in that situation. Adults are the ones who need the time outs and we need to be responsible enough to let others know when we need to take them.

I took time outs with my wife on occasion when we became frustrated with the pace at which the other one is doing something or when words were about to become volatile. There is no point to fighting with someone you love and this includes children. Give them something else to occupy their time with and then you as the responsible party take time for yourself. Everyone needs time to be alone and think. Do not be ashamed about it and do not ignore your mind.

RESPECT and TOUGH LOVE

There are many people in the world who are like myself and hate misbehaving or crying children. We hate to hear stories about them when we can do nothing about it. So please make your children behave and learn so that I/we can have a better life.

When a child refuses to learn or be respectful, it is too often that we slap a label on them such as Attention Deficit Disorder or Attention Deficit Hyper Disorder. The correct diagnosis in the vast majority of children who act out is more likely "parental neglect". We're too busy trying not to miss our favorite mind numbing television show or fighting about whose turn it is to do something to give children the love and attention they need. I submit that when you have a child you are entering into a contract. You have forfeited your rights to frolic about and be selfish for the next 18 years. You agree to spend every waking free moment actively loving your child.

This includes tough love. Lessons learned by tears and time. Impressions formed by a swatting hand. Don't be in an uproar about abuse if that is normally your torch. In my youth I was maybe hit a total of 6 or 7 times and I deserved every damn one of them. I learned not to bawl in a supermarket, not to steal, not to swear (remember I grew into TS at age 15-ish), not to be violent lest I face a power 100 times greater than my own. These are valuable lessons, which if you are smart you only have to learn and at the same time.

One problem we face today is that our children are involved in various degrees of crime. Of course there are more than enough adults who participate as well, but the majority of them did not just take it up late in life. They started when they became early teens. I do not have children nor do I plan to, so I suppose it is easier to express more radical views than the majority of parents would. Being a person of conviction though, you can believe that I would stand by my word on this as well as everything else I state.

I firmly believe that parents have become entirely too limp with the discipline and rule setting for their children. No longer do kids respect anything their parents' say. No examples are even necessary here. Kids do not have any fear of God or of serious retribution. I did not take up the conscience use of profanity until I was in high school (very late for males). I seriously thought that God would strike me down with a lightning bolt had I even a profane thought. Actually I believe it all stems back to the giving of "time outs" at an early age. "Time-out" is the biggest bunch of nonsense crap lack of responsibility I've ever heard of. Tough love is the thing that's missing with our children today.

Tough love means recognizing that someone you love has a problem they are not willing to resolve with you by means of a legitimate conversation. If you care enough about them and need closure of an issue, you need to set a precedent to establish authority. Issues we have in our lives are only resolved in a few ways. Direct confrontation hurts the most, however it is the most effective. I openly challenge anyone to make a case for another method that achieves results, positive or negative, better than confrontation. The other option is really to set back and let them run their own lives, completely. They will do it anyway so why are you trying to intervene? If you choose this method you have no grounds to offer advice, criticism, approval, or anything else. Understand? Without commanding at least respect, you have no platform on which to preach.

The tough part of tough love is not in the saying of words to your kids; it is in the standing of your ground. My parents had a unique perspective. They commanded respect and a whole lot more. They chose however the passive method to our rearing. They were very adamant about not offering advice on the girls we dated, the sports we played, the friends we had, anything. We made a lot of bad decisions as to the company we kept, but they let us make those choices and they supported everything. The interesting thing that happened was that every time we learned we were wrong, we also saw the strength and love it took our parents to let us do those things. This is still their philosophy today. Total support: as is evidenced by the fact that I was unemployed and chasing a dream for a long time. My mother will admit that my style stresses her out but she won't admit opinions on anything else.

There was one notable exception to this rule that actually had a much unexpected outcome. It involved a girl I was seeing who wanted me to get an earring. This was taboo. I vividly recall them saying "If you get an earring, do not come home!" Well I got one and went right home to dinner. They said it wasn't that bad and that was the end of it. I had pushed the envelope but not because I knew they wouldn't throw me out. I thought they would do that. I knew they would still love me; they just didn't want a freak on display in their house. (I think they thought I was going to get a dangling skeleton or death symbol of some kind. It was just a stud, but they were afraid because I had long hair.) I was ready to face having to move out. That was the law they laid down and I accepted it. Besides, I had just started getting sex on a regular basis for the first time. It always makes you think you're ready to move out.

DICIPLINE

This is just my personal opinion of course but as a part of tough love I believe that you should beat the living tar out of your kids when they do something wrong. I believe it should not only be allowed but also praised as being a part of responsible parenting. The only child I have is my beagle puppy, and when she does something wrong, the proverbial "hand of God" used to come down. I love my puppy and she loves me more than anything but between the two of us we cannot communicate with more than a handful of words, so other methods like kisses, petting and sometimes punishment have to be used. The same is true of children. I thank God that we don't have to go there anymore. I still feel bad about it and apologize to her every now and then. Life is good for us now!

Until kids have reached a certain level of development when something inherently tells them not to infuriate their parents, then you have to teach by method of consequences. Some children are more fortunate than others of course. I was hit a total of maybe 7 times in my adolescence. My ex-wife says she was never hit, but that doesn't mean she never deserved it. My father-in-law was just a very patient man. I have good patience skills but only with my girlfriend (when I have one) and Daisy.

Getting back to discipline though, there are things you can do to influence the behavior patterns of your children without being violent.

Removing all sense of privacy is one such (very effective) action. Take the doors away from their rooms. All of the doors. Dressers, bathrooms and closets if necessary. Why do they need to have doors anyway, unless they are doing something deviant? You don't want them to be a deviant, so that seems like a pretty damn good starting point which helps allow you to monitor their behavior.

From there you should continue as necessary to use sensory deprivation by removing television and phone privileges and establishing proper phone etiquette. If you do not want your children to hang out with hoodlums, then do not let them communicate like hoodlums with their friends.

Lay the smack down upon your children's asses until they are good. If they don't like your style of justice then let them leave to starve and fend for themselves and become nappy little parasites. Sever all communication. If you have done everything right as a parent and your child still misbehaves after all of that, then you just plain have a bad seed. What do you do with a bad seed? Do you nurture it and give it love and help it try to grow? No. Don't be a pathetic loser. You spit it out, sometimes smash or crush it under your heel and then throw it away which translates into one thing = Abortion in the 60th trimester. Thank you South Park™.

As a final note on discipline, I would encourage you to think of some cruel and unusual punishments which will require your child to think about their actions and the way they impact others. By doing this you will help them to realize at a younger age that life really does suck on another level than they even thought possible. That going to work every day is actually worse than school, and that they really do make your life a lot harder by not being good.

As a suggestion, volunteer your child's time and have them mow the school lawn, come in at 6:30 am with the lunch lady, put on a hair net and help out in the cafeteria. Maybe clean the locker rooms and stay until the janitor leaves at 7pm. Let them be made to clean up piss around toilets, repaint walls and grind away graffiti with a drill. Let the punishment fit the crime because it's cool and it has always, through out history, been the right thing to do.

TEENAGERS

The youth in America today tend to piss me off. There are two things that no one likes; a smart-ass and a non-conformist. They are labeled as such because they don't belong and in their current state of rebellion no one wants them. Why don't we just whip them back into shape? During my tenure as a fast food manager, I was privileged enough to hire two twin brothers. They were very tall and fairly strong high school football players. Their father made them go out and get part time jobs to learn respect. You could tell that he beat them at times growing up, but they were the nicest and most polite kids I have ever had the pleasure of meeting. They called me Sir all of the time because I was their boss. I referred to them as Sir because they earned my respect. We always had a good time within the boundaries of productive work and we made progress as a team because of their examples.

Beating your kids is OK! Just don't do it for sport or when you're drunk. You can go to hell for that, I'm pretty sure.

Just one more thing I want to add here real quickly about what you give your children when they are growing up. Parents need to be a whole lot more involved in everything they do. Let's take for example cell phones and texting nudie pictures. Sex-ting as they call it is not a problem. Sending pictures of your naked parts is actually a very cool idea. Sex-ting is awesome, but it is for adults. Your fat lazy children don't need phones. They don't need a Game Boy™. They need to learn how to interact with all the other personality types of the other children at school. They need physical activity.

My generation didn't have squat for phones. We didn't have pagers yet until 1998 or about then. If your kid wants a phone and starts to cry about it you punch them. That's pretty simple. Don't talk bull-shit to me about your child's fuckin' safety. Um, here's a thought; maybe you shouldn't have kids if you can't dedicate your life to their supervising them and providing proper one-on-one development. Don't be weak. Once you produce a child you are non-verbally signing away your rights to having your own life for 18 years. Too bad, you lose. Want a life? Don't make babies.

SCHOOL

Junior high is nothing more than a popularity breeding ground for high school. You don't retain anything. Just give your kids cool clothes and teach them how to stand up for themselves while remaining respectful. Teach them about sex. Show them how babies can destroy hopes, dreams and entire lives if you are not ready. High school is nothing more than prep school for life although it really isn't run that way. What I mean is, the classes that are taught don't have much practical application. I'll give you some examples:

Civics – (a required course) I don't remember anything past how the 3 houses of government basically work. I learned how a Bill gets turned into law from Schoolhouse Rock. That class needs to incorporate how the stock exchanges work and we need to start teaching against party lines.

Foreign Language – Excellent class, we need more of it. This needs to start as a mandatory class in Jr. High and be required for 6 years all the way through HS. For at least 4 years I want to see a different language taught EVERY DAY! Russian, Chinese, French, Spanish and Arabic. I choose these for 2 reasons. Kids need to break down their natural barriers of cross cultural fear early and be reminded of them constantly. Later in life multi-lingual persons are vastly superior. These persons also have less hatred and more understanding of the world in general. Specialty language could be chosen for the last 2 years.

Math – sucks cow balls. If your child likes it, great. Let 'em go wild with math electives. If they hate it, give 'em a set of wrenches so they learn metrics, teach them long division and them give 'em a hall pass so they don't have to stress about something they are pre-destined not to care about. Chances are they need encouragement with physical activity.

Dress Code – We need to teach children the importance of not being ugly. This is different for every child and their classmates should be forced to help not hinder. We all need a leg up and real advice about hair, face, teeth and most of all fatness. Should we not teach about real life?

Dating and Marriage – How is this not a class already? Classroom dating with coaches would be sweet! Teach them about divorce rates and custody. Teach the boogers about attention, affection, appreciation and actually planning things for your partner. Especially in H.S. where it is vitally important that you are able to recognize who is currently a loser -vs- who will be a loser in the future -vs- who will remain timelessly cool and who really does have the biggest cock in school.   → ME

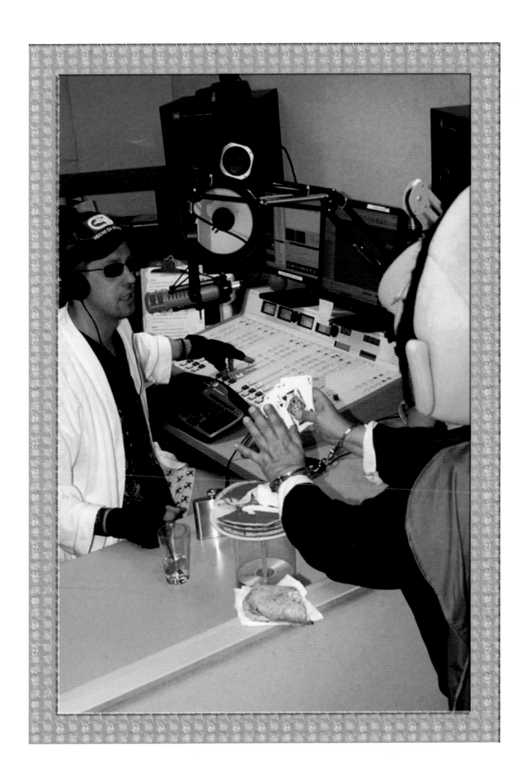

Air Play

Yes, it's the "Marshal" Douglas & Diaz show circa 1998 in Phoenix Arizona. Life was crazy back then. We drank and ate and had hookers in the studio. In this instance we were doing a remote in Las Vegas and Count Von Count was arrested for counting cards and taken to the county jail. She is attempting to explain the infraction and couldn't understand why the casino security would be suspicious.

When I get excited my hands used to sweat and I always had to go to the bathroom before going on the air. I drink margaritas or martinis on the air. All the greats do it. These are my luck beagle underwear from Target. Sometimes my girl comes in too. She's good and doesn't pee unlike Diaz. We were well on our way to setting up toilet microphones in the bathroom before somebody caught on and thought the better of it. Really though, everyone likes a certain amount of toilet humor. You can only play some Iron Butterfly or the long version of American Pie so many times when you have an emergency from all the damn coffee it takes to keep you awake at 7am. You go in at 4 but oddly enough you don't start really sagging until 7. Macarthur Park is another good long play tune.

See the computers in the back. Yeah, we didn't have those in the day. We had to stack up CD's about 20 high to make it for a while and you had to pull your own commercials from a spinning tape rack (they are called "carts" but they looked like 8-tracks) Same basic functions. Anyway, we rocked every single time we came on the air there was chaos and general destruction.

THE CHOSEN PATH

CHAPTER XI

CHILDHOOD

One of the very few complaints I have about the way I was raised was that we were told we could do and/or be anything that we wanted. I no longer believe this is true for me. If your parents are wealthy and live in the right city, only then is a child afforded the opportunity to choose their own destiny.

I am bitter every day because I inherently feel like I am owed something. I know I am not yet I just can't shake the feeling. It is bigger than I am. My spirit has a bigger potential than my body can handle. Perhaps it is a calling to do something more. There have been no big breaks for me though. I have to do everything myself. Every single time I rely on someone else I feel let down, so I have tried to stop asking.

I was robbed, plain and simple. I remember the point in time at which my father had decided to retire from the military. We were living in Omaha, Nebraska and I didn't particularly want to be there. I recall that when they were looking at houses in the area we were invited to give our input. That was a rouse to get us kids to shut up. We never really had an input option. I never saw our house before we moved in but it wouldn't have gotten my vote anyway so it didn't really matter. There was no beach, the weather was crappy, and even in the seventh grade I didn't see a lot of opportunity there for a bright future.

INCIDENCES OF YOUTH

As I see it my junior high and high school years were much less wild than everyone else's. This is speculation. Come to find out that after 2 reunions people apparently thought I had lots of fun. Who knew? In my perspective I really didn't cause a whole lot of trouble, and as a result I had doomed myself to never reach my potential popularity. We were raised very well mannered though, and I considered a lot of what the other kids were doing to be wrong. So I removed myself from a lot of situations. I can't speak for others, but I certainly saw myself as a gangly nerd with bad hair.

The only exception to this was my entire 5th grade year. I don't know what happened but I was a hellion. I must have hormonally changed really early because I had the school record for writing sentences. My two friends and I did everything from sneaking into the girls' bathroom and looking over the stalls, to bringing dirty magazines to school and looking at them on recess, to threatening children with grappling hooks made from paper clips, to spitting on kids from the monkey bars. When the three of us were punished for the magazine incident we caught the Principal doing some reading of her own when we walked into her office. There were bigger kids around but they never picked on me because we had a 13-year-old girl in our class. She had failed a few times. Anyway, she was big, smoked, tattooed herself with pens and happened to kind of like me.

I was really into girls. I remember Blondie had the #1 record in the country with *Heart of Glass* and I would have done anything to make it with Deborah Harry.

During high school and college I did a variety of things that I thought were original. We had a lot of fun and never got arrested. I had plenty of encounters with the police and the law to this day never seems to be on my side, but I get by. I think I ride the line of being considered a public nuisance and that doesn't help me. People with passion tend not to care about such things though.

Most of my High School graduating class was pretty lame and we had made it halfway through the year without any pranks having been performed at all. Therefore on January 3, 1988 my best friend Bob and I executed what was as masterful plan in grand design. It was original and genius. I have to give him credit for actually going along with this. Sometimes people can get injured whilst pulling off a good prank, right Bob? (I dropped a large tool on his head once but he survived).

Now being as it was cold enough to shrivel my "sack" while sitting next to a fire (-40 w/ the wind chill), we fell upon the idea that we should use nature's brute force to our advantage. It rarely snowed enough in Omaha for the board to call school off, so that was our clear goal. To become heroes in the eyes off all attendees by forcing the school to somehow give us the day off. Really the plan was brilliant. We would force the school to close for the day by shooting dirty old tap water into all of the locks and around all of the doorframes. If no one could enter the building, then were obviously not going to hold classes were we?

We set out after 12:10AM in my mother's car, which we parked two blocks away from the school so no one would notice. We were frozen by the time we even made it to the building. We were loaded with spray bottles and started hitting the locks.

They froze instantly and the water expanded so fast that ice came pushing back out of the keyholes. Then we would pour just enough around the door to make it difficult as well. We hit every single entrance that night including the garage doors to the maintenance room and the library fire exits which didn't even have outside handles.

The next morning was fun. I didn't have a first period anyway so I didn't have to be up, but my brother did. The reports from classmates all confirmed that they were not able to break into the school until 7:55am. Five minutes before classes started, and then only through one door. We were only cheated from victory because the whore-bitch school Superintendent had decided it was a better idea to forcibly enter the school than to just write off one simple day and let us have our moment. Apparently first they tried a blowtorch, which melted the water but also the grease inside the locks turning the grease into a gluey substance and still preventing the use of keys. At this point, being really pissed off they destroyed the locks with drills and other tools.

At this point they were in the main entrance and could push open the other doors from the inside so the kids would have school. They couldn't wait for the sun to naturally and slowly melt the rest of the ice away, no. They felt it imperative to destroy every lock on the premises like they were freeing slaves instead of holding them. Dense huh? Conceptually, a high percentage of people in the Midwest should just go ahead and have sex with cows, because the level of intelligence in the person they are creating is just not there. I believe I already covered this.

OK, so stupidity reigns over all the country, my apologies to the Midwest. We all know more than our share of persons who are ridiculously stupid.

So what was the verdict? How did the other students rate our stunt? Well before I can tell you that, I am inclined to mention that we did face minor justice. You see, most people (out of boredom) are inherently nosey. Even though we had undertaken our mission in the middle of the night on a night when no human should have been out, apparently some nosey neighbor whose life was bad enough to not sleep had gone out for a drive or something and noticed a different car on their street. (We never got a clear answer on how this happened). Well, they reported to the police that there was a suspicious vehicle outside and had taken the license number. The next day when they found out what had happened to the high school, I guess they ran the car plates and found it was registered to my brother. He had plausible deniability and didn't know a thing, so when they called him into the office and raked him across the coals, he was a bit distraught. The only thing he could do was to suggest that either my mother was out or that I had taken the car.

Well when they finally called Bob and me into the office, we freely admitted that we did it, which immediately through them into a loop. They couldn't figure out why two good students would do such a thing. They didn't even grasp the notion of a senior prank, and they refused to believe that we only used water. The Principal swore to almighty God that we used super glue or something else. The students all thought it was awesome and even thanked us for trying. A year later I can even recall seeing a girl named Michelle from our class on the college campus. She was with two of her friends, but she stopped to tell us that she had heard about what we did and she thought it was cool. Michelle was a stone cold fox and that was all the complement we needed at the time.

(Note to future generations, we did pay a fine of $80+ dollars each for lock replacement and received 3 days off). Going forward, we were never implicated in anything else and are much to deviant to be stopped by a license plate and a nosy neighbor.

Later pranks included stealing street signs, running yarn balls through a house under construction with no walls, smashing numerous things in front of trains, and erecting our own street sign (which lasted on a prominent cornet for a month). People couldn't handle merging at that intersection so it read, "MOVE IT! Use the extra lane you paid for (unless you're from Iowa)."

I think the event that opened the throttle on my true rowdy nature was throwing a bachelor party for my friend Trevor when we were 19 or so. Until then I was pretty tame. I also worked like a dog and was too involved with swimming and music to do much else. At any rate, Trevor decided to marry fairly young which I thought was great. So I threw him a party in the soon to be abandoned house of my friend Bob. At the height there might have been 40 people there, so it wasn't too large, but we completely destroyed everything. We broke windows, knocked the porch over, had a bean burrito fight, it was pretty ugly. Chicks came and stole our booze but we were already too far-gone to stop it. I ended the night falling down the stairs because I couldn't get my pants back up after going pee. Other friends Mike and his fiancée Jenna in particular found me that way. I didn't have a whole lot of shame left after that one.

COLLEGE

I have more memories of the mind numbing cold in Nebraska than of anything else. At the University of Omaha, the wind is always in your face, never at your back. Amazing but true. There's no pretty snow to go along with it either, just the freezing cold.

So I started as a music performance major, and worked that for two years until I realized that I was headed for opera. I love classical works and had a good time singing them but it wasn't the career choice for me. I wanted to still have something to do with music and so I turned to broadcasting and radio. (I do hold a B.A. in Broadcast Production and I actually have a reel-to-reel machine and can edit tape. Punk fuckers now just use computers. The hate flows through me.)

So I drank more than my share at this stage, unbeknownst to many. The same friend Mike and I actually belonged to a small group that we called the Heavy Drinkers Club (more on this in the next chapter). I put it there because it is all about enjoying or destroying your life. The initiation was a little rough, which is why it was a small group. Mike and I skipped out of class all the time to go to our favorite bar Sharky's, and then we would blow 8 dollars on video games in the kids arcade while we were still drunk. We showed up to music appreciation class frequently smelling like beer and nachos. People really told us this, but it was an unbearable no-credit yet required class.

I had a few fun classes like archery/badminton, film history, and physics of life. As I mentioned I took that astronomy course with the professor who told us alien factoids most of the time. He was cool. Mostly I stared at the breasts of my female classmates, when coats didn't cover them up.

I SHOT THE TRANSMITTER

Well, almost. So I'm on the air one night at a radio station I worked for in the 90's and the guy who was running the AM station down the hall was an avid gun collector. He'd bring them in all the time. He even loaded his own ammo. One day I brought in my Ruger .45 for show. It was a nice gun and being from Nebraska I had shot off several hundred rounds before; just messing around being drunk and bored at night, so I knew what I was doing also. We took the magazine out and pulled back the slide just to make sure it is safe like you normally would. Mind you, the AM guy is a gun PRO! Somehow we both missed one bullet that was lodged inside that had come loose from the clip. It was destiny I guess. Fortunately I was pointing at the floor when I pulled the trigger.

The gun went off very close to both the transmitter and my foot. I thought I hit it because we couldn't hear anything. After crapping my pants just a little and thinking I was going straight to jail we realized that we just couldn't hear because the gun went off in an 8' x 8' padded room. I'm still on the air at this point so we are writing each other "holy crap" notes on paper and decided we still have to go live and do our breaks without being able to hear. (There is a small chance that Tequila may have been involved also.) We would just use the clocks and count down the time remaining in the songs intro. It worked but the studio reeked of gunpowder, so we still needed a cover story lest we go to jail in the morning.

Randy was a smoker as are most DJ's and he was always walking by my booth to go outside when he had a long song playing. The station was actually moving to another building in about 2 weeks so he figured it would only be a minor slap on the wrist if they thought we were smoking in the booth. Little did they know he was about to do some chain smoking and blow right into the foam on the walls, so Randy did his part. If they asked about the hold in the carpet I was going to tell them that I had no choice and I had to bring my dog in that night; she had chewed a small hole that I was totally willing to pay for. After all of that it turns out that absolutely nobody cared. They never asked us any questions and we never did find the bullet!

BECOMING AN ENTREPRENEUR

There came a point in my life where I decided I could no longer stand to listen to anybody. Even the news and newspapers are virtually useless to me. All that they had to say was a bunch of crap and it was never anything valuable like the inside track on a real job. I discovered early on that I could learn to do almost any given job, and after 3 months time I would do it better than the boss. This led me to many job changes just to combat the intense boredom that comes from repetition. It also raised a lot of frustration inside. This trend would continue through my career in radio as ridiculously under-qualified individuals continued to beat me out for jobs. I began to notice a lack of vision on the part of employers. If my ideas didn't match their own (really lame ideas) then I was surely wrong. It takes a big person and an open mind to listen to employee's suggestions. Employers also have a need to cover their own backs so to speak. Indeed, why would you want to hire somebody that may in fact become future competition? Wouldn't it be better to hire somebody who is not on the same level as you? Job security is good but in this case it does reek of cowardice.

In October of 1997 I was released from a job as promotions coordinator at a top 40 station where I had worked for 2 years. At the point of my termination, I was one of the best known, liked and respected men in town with that job. I worked hard at it, was made to put up with a lot of crap and ignorance, but I still did a damn good job.

Now Arizona is a "right to work" state which means that your employer can let you go without notice, severance or a reasonable explanation. When I was released I of course asked for a reason and I was told "We can't tell you, but I am really sorry". Fortunately I did respect the 2 men above me and knew that it was not their decision. The next part is purely speculation, but I figure I made too many waves and knew too much about the shifty practices of the upper management. There was a rumor though that the V.P. had video footage of the owner with little boys and that was why he always got his way, no matter how absurd it was.

I was happy to see that in the following weeks nearly every promotion failed and my replacement crashed the station van right out of the gate. I took a hiatus from radio for the next year. Later I founded *WaveFM.com* which was one of the first Internet-based radio stations.   I intended to start a revolution. Turns out we couldn't make any money with it. Its funny how after 15 years Internet radio still hasn't progressed into a legitimate business. It's become a hobby and a tax write off for companies like Yahoo.

After that I had no motivation left since I was now single and had no faith left in the system of working hard to get somewhere in life. It was then that I began to write this book but also that I put together a business plan. I had decided that the only way to get what I wanted would be to own a real radio station. Then I could do it all. Freedom to speak my mind, notoriety and attention, I could perform music, travel, meet people, and just have fun.

BROKERS

It didn't work out but I got so close!

Everyone who is frustrated will inevitably try to go into business for themselves at one point in their lives. That is the nature of things. We all think that we can do something better. Now many times a person encounters the need to acquire an existing business, or the funds needed to begin the venture. This is where the broker comes in and it was at this point that all of my proposals failed. I had money lined up and a great plan. I even found the perfect station to buy in Las Vegas. Once word got out about what I was trying to do, a conglomerate contacted my broker and worked me straight out of the deal. They just threw money at the problem (me) until I was out. Sucks hairy balls is what it does.

The majority of brokers in any field are not really concerned with the success of your project, but rather they are in it for the quick scam. Make the money and then leave town. I say to you now that any legitimate services broker will only collect a fee after you have gotten whatever it is that you want. They will also never charge you a retainer fee because they will be more than confident in their own abilities to get the job done for you.

I have decided, through great research and a lot of money that business brokers are essentially people who couldn't get it done for themselves. These are all scum. Most of them have their own dreams or ideas about business that they would like to start. They invested the same time and money that I did only to lose on all accounts. Rather than accepting defeat and moving forward or trying to help someone else by utilizing their knowledge of what does not work, they would try to recoup their own personal loses on the backs of another who would just be beginning the journey.

They are scum. They prey upon the idealistic. Do not trust anyone who claims to be a money broker. Now there are many types of brokers. Whether you are looking for a house or a business as was I, never contract the services of anyone who would require a retaining fee. I cannot stress that enough. If they are confident, they will not need funds to support them for any period of time more than 2 weeks. Most honestly successful brokers have a dedicated circle of persons with whom they have worked before. All they need do is place a 10-minute phone call to the right pre-selected person and your deal is done. Oddly, the field of literary agency is much the same.

CURRENTLY

If I can lay around for 8 months and not do crap if I want to, then that is success. By the same token, if I can work 20 hours but get paid like I was working 60 then that is also a win. Understand?

"Success is measured by how much work I do NOT HAVE TO do."

So how exactly do retired people have the right to be bored anyway? You can always learn a new language, play an instrument or donate your time to a good cause. I hear people say that and it's just ridiculous to me. I have 4 working passions at this point in my life. Now that I have finished this book, I can die in peace but these are the projects that I will move on to in my spare time.

1) __The Creative Minds Foundation__ is a project that I would like to re-start in order to help people that have trouble effectively communicating and cooperating in society. Being one such person and having received no help, it is something that I am compelled to do. The foundation would seek to help individuals that have or think that they have brilliant ideas; to either realize their dreams or to direct them in such a manner that their ideas be refined into a workable solution. If they are deemed to be unworkable then they can be laid to rest by a jury of their peers. The IRS tells me that this is not a tax deductible cause and doesn't actually qualify for exempt status. I don't care. You can still donate money to a cause you believe in. I might just have to base it out of another country where smart people are in charge.

2) __Performing:__ I want to do things with my personality in many different aspects. Performance is one of the few things in life that gives me a natural high and it's the only thing work related that I enjoy. Here's a short list of the things I want to do now.

- Get back on the air; radio and TV, film, voice-over a cartoon character. Moreover, one that is extremely powerful and possibly robotic in some manner. I won't work with bad animation though. I am producing some screen plays. One is a comedy to go hand-in-hand with this stupid book and the other is a science-fiction work requiring massive amounts of collateral, which I alone do not have. I did some work as the 1st Technical and Sound Director for Bob's Big Monster Movie _SACRIFICE_.

- Play in a 9 piece band on board a cruise ship and record one hell of a good album with my some of my songs on it.

3) _**Invest in a Restaurant/Bar**_ I only want to do this so I can go to a place where I don't get charged for anything. I want to have the best establishment in the world where everyone wants to go. The travel channel will even recommend it. It will have all the crucial elements of a total class outfit including places to sleep if you're to wasted, hot tubs to have dinner in and lots of tight young naked girls running around rubbing or kissing me and calling me Poppa. That's not too bad is it? _Poppa's_ will be decorated with palm trees, have skylights, food that really does make you orgasm and feature live jazz musicians. Maybe even a conference room for working professionals.

4) _**Leaving America Trading Co.**_ is just a simple idea for an online store. It will only showcase cool things and will not sell junk. Stainless steel rings, great music from unknown artists and great original t-shirts will be some of the offerings. I would like to get an import license so I can bring in some fantastic Rum to the states. This is just something to show my general contempt for authority in a somewhat public and ongoing setting as if the book

isn't enough. I'll do this when and if I get bored with the other stuff. It's in the pipeline though.

For an up to date, accurate listing of all my projects, please visit
www.dpmedia.org

IN SUMMARY

I attract horribly disfigured women who are the biggest victims on the planet. I have worse than bad luck. I could never get a really good job because people were too afraid of what I might do. My body aches from several not at fault accidents. I am very talented and exceptionally kind however normal women think that this is a front and so they run away. Things are getting better every day. Seriously, I just want to live in peaceful solitary...being married with a puppy, playing music, making others happy and helping where I can.

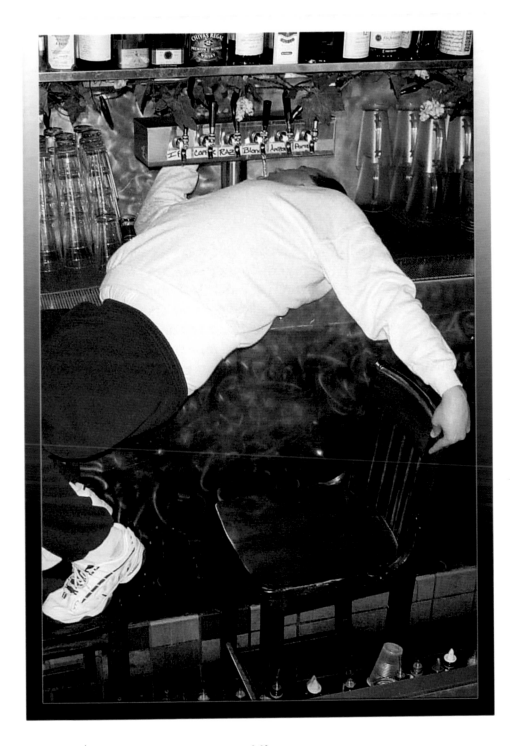

"FATMAN FANTASY"

A photo about what every man in his most basic state would like to do. Drink with reckless abandon straight from the tap. It is not about being a fat man or even being slobbish. It is not even about drinking beer. It could be Cool-aid for that matter. This man is going after something he loves regardless of the physical pain involved to get it!

The photo was taken for comedic value alone. Men do not need glasses to enjoy themselves nor do they even need to be vertical. The fact that the beer is flowing onto his clothing and the floor indicates that men in a primal moment of enjoyment do not really care about much at all. Ironically, none of these things matter in the real world either. If one were to pull such a stunt in a public bar, would it be a big matter to applaud and then just clean it up? Would any harm be done if he was not punished and did not go to jail?

This was the first picture that I ever took for this book. I did take on what now would be considered on old school digital camera. I think the pixel count was 2.3 but I loved it.

Date Taken: 7.26.2001

Location: Tucson, AZ by the campus

Model: Roy M.

Camera: Sony DSC-P50. ISO 400.

THEORIES and the SECRET of LIFE

CHAPTER XII

Every one who knows me will tell you that I have a theory for nearly everything. If I do not, then the subject hasn't been of concern long enough for me to formulate one. If you give me a few minutes though, I would create one for you. We'll get to these in just a few minutes.

Plain and simple the secret to life is to be happy. God (however you perceive God to be) can experience joy vicariously through us. This is why we were created. So that God may feel even more joy. Joy can come through any number of experiences for us such as smelling a flower, enjoying great coffee in the morning and swimming in the ocean or even watching your favorite television show. It doesn't matter what you do to find it, only that you recognize the value of it and take the time to thank God for giving you that opportunity in life to experience joy.

Live your life as if you were on screen in a movie, where you are the main character and everything you do affects the outcome of the plot. When you look at something like a woman's body or a flower or a landscape or a building in a city, look at it through the perspective of a high definition lens that allows you to see the minutest details at every angle that you wish to view. Life is beautiful that way. We should all live that way, and be the hero of the story. Be important when you think you are nobody!

CARPE DIEM / SEIZE THE DAY

Life is a bowl of surprises. There are those who will tell you that a person makes their own successes or failures. This is true, but only to a degree. There are many workings of the world that we do not understand. Blind and dumb luck account for many of the successful people we know of today. Scams and deceit also make up a large portion. Of course you can't forget parental influence (the worst kind of achieved success).

"Everything happens for a reason". How many times have you wanted to whop someone's ass for saying that? The more appropriate phrase would be "Everything happens as a result of something else". If you take water from the well, someone later will go thirsty. If you neglect to give love to your spouse, someone else will try. If you are an illegal alien with no insurance driving a stolen car and you get in an accident with a law abiding citizen, you'll not only create a life crisis for probably a really nice person but you'll also not face any real punishment here in America just because we love you and value your illegality.

Is it fair? Absolutely not. Is it true? Absolutely.

My point is that you should not focus on the negative; I have done that for you. Simply realize why bad things happen and then try to get out of the way when they are about to. All of life is connected. Until I am elected high evolutionary decision maker for the planet, there will always be a Yang for every Yin. When I am though, punishment will reign down from above and good will win 90% of the time. The white space will dominate!

There are many steps to take in learning to truly enjoy life:

1. Do not fear death. You should still act sensibly, but know that when your spirit leaves its temporary shell, you will be much happier.

266

2. Learn to appreciate and enjoy your food. Make noises when you eat. Let the cook know how much you love what they have done for you.

3. Express your love for those people who have it every chance you get without hesitation or shame. You should be envious of people who have mastered this goal. You have to know they get hurt a lot and they keep moving forward.

4. Marvel at the wonder of creation and everything you are able to experience with all your senses; no matter how many you have remaining.

5. Give until it hurts and then relax. Just watch your seeds grow. Don't be too prideful of yourself.

6. Practice transcending in one of its many forms.

7. Tell both of your parents you love them. I have found immense joy in this.

8. Practice giving genuine compliments to complete strangers without wanting anything in return.

9. Be spontaneous. Never make excuses for why you cannot do something. Act out, have fun, and most importantly try the things you never thought you could do. Get away from what you know and travel to a third world country. You will be a better person when you return.

10. Be decisive. Even if it means that someone else would make a different decision or that you'll sometimes be wrong.

It takes a lot of power and a lot of focus just to wake up early every morning, to make a list of goals and accomplish them all. I salute everyone who competes in the cold cruel world. People who perfect their bodies without steroids and who sharpen their minds impress me. I look pretty good but I have my Three-Toed Sloth moments every day. I would be doing better if I didn't lose time to napping every day and staring at the wall.

HONESTY

Honesty is the hallmark of every great person. More often misunderstood than accepted. It commands respect from others who practice it. It goes ignored and unappreciated by those who don't.

To practice honesty can be brutal to both sides of an interaction. We have come to a point in our male / female relationships where an honest compliment invokes several negative responses. That's not a good thing.

Feelings of estrangement, fear, loathing, and disgust should not be what you experience after a receiving a compliment. It might not be the unwarranted "come on" that you think it is. Women need to go to school to become better judges of character. Nice guys don't deserve to be bastardized for your prior mistakes. When a compliment is delivered with sincerity and emotion it should be recognized and appreciated for the amount of courage and integrity it takes to present.

The receiving end of a genuine compliment is an uncomfortable situation particularly if it comes from an acquaintance that is less than desirable to you.

Compliments only come my way in one of two varieties. The first is approval of performance for my music, a job, or intimacy. The second and vastly rarer of the two is for my appearance. I have no problems with compliments about performance of anything I do. The general rule with compliments about appearance is that all the men in my family strangely attract unearthly large women somewhere in the sedan weight class. It is hard to accept these even though they are very genuine. This is where choosing not to date on the whole tends to save me. I need to learn how to say "I really like you; however you are a sedan and although you have a 4 star crash rating you are still too much solid mass for my weak back to handle".

The situations may vary for you but whatever they are try to be honest when you reply. <u>Honest and diplomatic.</u>

Tip 1. Preface every negative response with a buffer statement. Usually "Thank you" at the onset of the reply sets a tone of acknowledgment and respect. They cannot legitimately hate you for what you are about to say if they respect you. They can illegitimately hate you but then it's not your problem.

Tip 2. Don't sugar coat it. For the sake of God or whatever power you believe in do not ever do this again. How is the person you are letting down ever to learn anything about themselves or how to correct their problems if you do not tell them what they are.

Tip 3. Make a small gesture of physical contact. Grab and hold a finger. Touch their shoulder. Look into their eyes. This let's them know you're still human even though you appear to be an ogre and you will feel their plight as well. You will learn from the experience also and that's what counts.

Tip 4. Try not to hesitate.   The complimentor can smell uneasiness. It does not support the respect angle.

SAYINGS TO LIVE BY
(That are actually worth something)

These are just cool little bits of conversations that I have remembered because they can actually apply to real people. I have recently noticed that there are entire books and several calendars published about noteworthy sayings, but I just wanted to give you a few of my personal favorites. Here they are: If I knew who quoted it first I would give them credit. I am telling you that I don't know.

I'll put the ones I think you may have heard before toward the end of the list, so that you will be more impressed with the potentially new ones.

"It is better to be a big ass fish in a big ass pond." - Me

Never look for a worm in the apple of your eye.
(Langston Hughes I believe)

"Success seems to be largely a matter of hanging on when others have let go." - William Feather (I don't know who he is.)

Two wrongs most definitely do make a right.

If your ship doesn't come in, swim out to it. If you're not a good swimmer then consider yourself marooned.

Be nice to other people, they outnumber you six billion to one.

The people around you were placed on Earth for your amusement, so don't hesitate to laugh.

"Knowledge is knowledge, not power, but it does make you look good." - Me

Work like you don't need the money,
Love like you've never been hurt.
And dance like nobody is watching.

"There's no room for TEAM in the word I" - Me
(Smoke that in your motivational pipe)

Forget your past or the future may forget you.

You miss 100% of the shots you never take.

Never say never unless you intend to bet.

Cold hands, warm heart. – (Very true of me!)

Love is like war; easy to begin but hard to stop.

Why buy the cow when you can get the milk for free.

THINGS TO SEE BEFORE YOU DIE

Well you can't physically go to see all of the seven Wonders of the Ancient World because only one of them still remains. This information was found on the Internet under the website http://ce.eng.usf.edu/pharos/wonders. They are in chronological order:

1) **THE GREAT PYRAMID OF GIZA** - A gigantic stone structure near the ancient city of Memphis, serving as a tomb for the Egyptian Pharaoh Khufu.

2) **THE HANGING GARDENS OF BABYLON** - A palace with legendary gardens built on the banks of the Euphrates River by King Nebuchadnezzar II.

3) **THE STATUE OF ZEUS AT OLYMPIA** – 353 B.C. an enormous statue of the Greek father of gods, carved by the great sculptor Pheidias. Moved to Constantinople before being lost to a fire.

4) **THE TEMPLE OF ARTEMIS AT EPHESUS** - A beautiful temple in Asia Minor erected in honor of the Greek goddess of hunting and wild nature.

5) **THE MAUSOLEUM AT HALICARNASSUS** - A fascinating tomb constructed for King Maussollos, Persian satrap of Caria. Stood for only 16 years and was toppled by earthquake.

6) **THE COLOSSUS OF RHODES** - 282 BC a colossus of Helios the sun god, erected by the Greeks near the harbor of a Mediterranean Island. Stood for 56 years but was destroyed by earthquake.

7) **THE LIGHTHOUSE OF ALEXANDRIA** - A lighthouse built by the Ptolemies on the island of Pharos off the coast of their capital city.

It was the Greeks who composed this original list and so it is easy to understand that many of the places edifices stemmed from Greek culture. The physical limitations of their world were small however, and so they were unaware of other potential wonders such as the **Great Wall of China** that existed in their same time line.

What you can do is make it a point in your life to go and see the most fascinating and remarkable things that the modern world has to offer. Even attempting to see a few of these wonders will enhance your lives forever. There are lists of some Forgotten, Modern and Natural Wonders, which can be found and studied on many different websites. The Natural Wonders list is currently being worked on.

If a new list is put together it should hold true to form and the wonders should have to be the true engineering marvels of our time. We are in the industrial age so I don't agree with the choices that were made. I agree that they are spectacular but should be retiled as remaining wonders of the ancient world. You'll see what I mean.

On 07/07/2007 a new list of still standing 7 Modern Day, Man-Made Wonders of the World was released to the public. They are also in chronological order:

1) **THE GREAT WALL OF CHINA** - Construction started around 220 B.C. Called the "10,000 Li Long Wall". The only man made structure visible from space. In the northern region, beginning at the coast not far from Peking. At one time it spanned 4233 miles long.

2) **PETRA** - Building began around 9 B.C. A city carved into the sandstone rock in the country of Jordan. Founded by the Nabataea Arabs it was seen as a site of great commercial and military importance. It was successfully defended against 3 empires many times until finally falling under Roman control circa 100AD.

3) **THE ROMAN COLOSSEUM** - Italy 70 – 82 A.D. The Amphitheater stands virtually in the middle of the city and

all the various events that took place there were tributes of sort to the Roman empire.

4) **THE PYRAMIDS AT CHITCHÉN ITZÁ** - Pre-800 A.D. A Mayan city composed of many temples with a central pyramid having been erected for Kukulkan, the "sovereign plumed serpent". Yucatan Peninsula, Mexico.

5) **MACHU PICCHU** - is the name of the mountain in Peru that this city in the clouds was built on by Emperor Pachacútec Circa 1460 A.D. It was most likely abandoned by the Incas following a small pox outbreak when the Spanish invaded. It was rediscovered only in 1911.

6) **THE TAJ MAJAL** - Built in Agra, India by Emperor Shah Jahan in the loving memory of his wife, Mumtaz Mahal. This marble and jewel inlaid wonder is the representation of everything a beautiful woman is put into architecture.

7) **STATUE OF CHRISTO RENEDOR** - Translated "Christ the Redeemer". Inaugurated in 1931 as a joint effort by the President and the Cardinal of Brazil. It took Brazilian designer Heitor da Silva Costa and French sculptor Paul Landowski 5 years to complete the work. The 38-meter statue of Christ the Redeemer stands 2000 feet above the hedonistic but beautiful city of Rio de Janeiro on Corcovado Mountain.

If you follow wrestling on television, I believe they dubbed both Andre the Giant and Chyna as wonders as well.

Other noteworthy ancient sites of our time would include:

THE MOAI STATUES OF RAPA NUI - Some 200+ volcanic rock-carved heads line the island, which once had a flourishing culture. The purpose of the statues is unknown. Easter Island, Chile

IGLESIA DE LA SAGRADA FAMILIA - The uncompleted masterwork church and tomb of architect Antonio Gaudi that lies in Barcelona, Spain. The project is spectacularly intricate and took over 40 years of his life. It may never be finished.

THE EIFFEL TOWER - Built for the 1889 World's Fair in Paris, France. It stood for some time as the tallest building in the world and is still revered as the representation of Europe.

ABU SIMBEL TEMPLE - Meant to unite the north and south of Egypt for King Ramses. The famous 4 statues watched the entrance.

ANGKOR WAT - Taking over 30 years to build in the 12th century, the world's largest temple is located in Cambodia. It was dedicated to the Hindu God Vishnu and symbolized the Hindu cosmos.

ALHAMBRA - Granada, Spain holds Europe's most visited tourist site. The palace sits on 13 hectares of land and was once converted into the royal residence of King Mohammed I. The grounds currently showcase an actual fortress, miniature coliseum, church, several residence buildings and stunning gardens.

PSALMS OF EL GRAN AMANTE

This little section contains wisdom and sayings that were inspired by meditations, hard times, and moments of reflection. <u>The words here are my own</u>. That is why I have called them Psalms instead of putting them with the sayings above that I cannot take credit for. Use the Lutheran chanting tones to sing them. I would hope that someone out there could benefit from what I have realized and use it to help them in their own lives. These are my songs of knowledge just as King David wrote the book of Psalms intended for worship. Mine are admittedly less prophetic.

1:1   Clarity is a means by which we should not only judge precious stones, but our lives.

2   We attain struggles by our greed; if we choose to learn and be wise we can be free of both.

3   As time waits for no one man, the only thing that transcends our time is the ignorance of mankind. Your mind has the ability to transcend its' self, and can remove negatives from your own life.

4   Balance is the key that separates one who has mastered life from the rest of us; they distinguish the harmony in the home and the chaos that lies outside, and one does not affect the other.

5   Failure although painful inspires growth. To continue to grow one must fail and then learn how not to.

6   Boredom stems from too much imagination and too little means. Give a man with boredom the means and you may watch the world change.

7   When interviewing; always assess a company worth by the quality of toilet paper it offers.

8   Patience and Testosterone have an inverse relationship. You can't have both.

9   Every individual on the earth is insignificant but unto themselves. It is only in great sacrifice or in loving service that we become important to the world.

10   There is a right and a wrong answer to every question, only the bias of the asker determines which is which.

11   Love can be bought, often for cheaper than you think.

PROVERBS

If a man tosses a ball into the sea, it will come back to him always on the crest of a wave. In like manner, when a man puts a good deed out into the world and seeks no reward, it will come back to him on the crest of many other good things.

Who is the bigger fool, the man who pours his soup from the bowl to his mouth, or the man who will use a spoon? All efforts are to savor the drop. Neither is the better.

If the good deeds of your life can all be written, then you have not done enough.

To be in wanting for things is to be misled in one's life. The purpose of work is solely of a sustaining nature. Personal gain with physical things is no gain at all in the continued development of the soul.

A good proverb is (not amazingly) a very tough thing to compose. You try writing a few and then ask someone else what they think of yours. Do you have the inner strength and harmony it takes or are you just a sad little weekend critic? Bite me eternally...

**The preceding proverbs were conceived in the mind of myself; Dón Párroco without assistance or reference from other materials. I will not here explain the meanings within, rather I would have others discuss them and upon learning their meanings hold them dear and pass them on as with other religious passages. I would like to include one other longer writing that I penned after spending some solitude in the woods: 6/13/06

Among the plants on earth, there are none that should be considered weeds and none should be pulled from the garden. Some plants will grow more quickly than others and some will be more visually appealing, but all have a place on God's Earth. In like manner treat all persons and living things including those whom you consider are or are not your brethren.

You should not destroy, demean or pick from the garden a person who does not fit into what you believe is right. One does not know unless one is God who should look or act the way they do and only God's plan is correct. Do you pretend to be able to do a better job than he who created the universe?

Do not cast them out, as they have equally as much birthright onto the world and all places in it as do you. This includes the home that you live in, which belongs to God alone as well. So make open your doors to all and receive the blessings that come from an open mind and spirit.

I do not say that this will not be a hard task. Do not feel a failure if it takes more than 1 lifetime for you to learn. I know this is the way, yet I have trouble adopting it myself as humbly I admit that man by its inherent sin nature is cruel.

VIRTUES and SINS

It's always nice to have handy a list of the things that you can and can't do; so here they are. Just for the record there is a freaky but interesting movie entitled *"Seven"* about this subject.

The Seven Holy Virtues	The Seven Deadly Sins
Faith	Lust
Hope	Envy
Charity	Sloth
Prudence	Pride
Justice	Avarice (Greed)
Temperance	Gluttony
Fortitude (Patience)	Anger

THEORIES

HERE THEY ARE!!! As you will notice, most of my theories relate to something I'm having a tangent about.

Theory of Similar Dysfunction - Let's say for example a woman is having a problem with vaginal dryness. She in her mind will blame the men she's with for not turning her on. She could be kind and use KY Jelly. A man who has an impotency problem will blame the woman he's with for not doing something right to turn him on. He could now take Viagra. My theory is that the reason most of their respective parts don't work right is because of over-use or mis-use. I don't think they should be allowed to use these products without having first to deal with someone of the similar dysfunction. Imagine it; she screams, "Oh my God, that hurts, you don't even know what you're doing!" then he shouts, "You're dryer than a plaster wall down here, you drinking water or eating paste?" They are perfect for each other and thus will help one another to grow. The same would be true for say a bigoted, self-centered hunk of a man to become stuck somewhere with a big-hearted, retarded minority but super hot female with only 1 leg. Sweet justice! The list could go on...

Theory of Impending Sales - For every idea that exists and for every item that is produced, there is a buyer. There may not necessarily be a tremendous market for the product or even a need by anyone to buy it. This theory states that people feel the overwhelming desire to obtain things. It could be anything just to make them feel better. If you put it out there someone will buy it. The key to the success of an individual item is the scale to which it is made readily available to the public. The more you put out, the more they will buy. The smart entrepreneur must know how to realize when saturation has occurred so they can take their money and proceed on to a new venture. The proof of this amazing theory is in the evidence of the sales of rap and heavy metal music. This stuff is straight-on crap yet it sells like hot tamales in a border town. So for anyone who has ever had an idea about a new product or invention; good luck and don't let anyone discourage you. Just take some marketing courses and do your homework. I am right about this and you know it.

Theory of Planned Obsolescence Absolution - The Theory of Planned Obsolescence says that if you engineer something to break down after a given period of time you thereby establish need and create demand. My theory says that if you corporate fuckers build something to break that I pay damn good money for, then you should have to fix it eternally for free. So build it right the first time and make this practice, obsolete or I will absolutely kick your ass! *P.S. - RIGID™ power tools suck donkey balls!*

Theory of Detachment Duality Reality - The Theory of Detachment says that the more a person wants something, the less it will come to them. You should exhibit a degree of detachment or otherwise you will drive yourself crazy. Additionally, my theory states that there inevitably exists two parts to the wanting and the achieving of anything; this is the duality. The first part is an insatiable desire to have whatever it is that you want and a never say die attitude. The second part is money. You have to be born with it, know somebody that has it or do something illegal to get it. In this second part also lies the reality factor. No matter how hard you want anything, you will not get it without money. The only exception and I mean only, is the love that two butt-rank ugly people are able to find in the flat bed portion of a truck in the woods.

Theory of Genial Development at Conception - I have this theory about making babies. I believe that it is possible, however not often done to change the physical composition that your baby will likely possess by changing your body or mind at the time of conception. If you both are pasty white people, then you should make every effort to be nice and tan for once in your life. If you are fat then have it sucked out. Correct your vision and have permanent laser hair removal done on any undesirable place. Fix everything in your power that is wrong with the both of you and then give your bodies a few weeks to heal and (I suspect) to re-write your genetic codes. Then try to conceive. The result will be a not so pasty child.

Theory of Obsessive Role Support Dichotomy - Do you clean the house before the maid comes over? Do you do your hair before you go to the beauty shop? Why? Is it because you want to be nice to them or is it because you are strange? This theory states that persons who exhibit such behaviors do not believe that anyone can accomplish the task as well as they can, so the effort is put forth to exemplify how they would like it to be done. These people are not the brilliant communicators they believe themselves to be. Why would they bother paying for the service to be performed after they have already begun the task?   The result is only to reveal their own inadequacies that they just worked so hard to hide.

Theory of Freaks - If more than 3 people at any particular gathering say that you are a freak, then you are. That is the rule and law. Perception is reality. You cannot fight or change it. You can only accept that you have been voted a freak and go home to change your ways.   This applies in particular to the certain religious sects in our culture.   If two more people are brave enough to publicly call you a bunch of freaks then you should all go home and just give it up, but you can continue if you really want to and if you don't mind the harassment.

Theory of Un-even Load - This theory is complementary to the previous in that there will be exceptions to that rule. There exist higher evolved beings as well as religiously developed persons who strive not to do wrong and always to help others and to love unconditionally. Bad things occasionally happen to these people as part of the un-even load because they are not the norm. In other words, there is so much negativity in the world that the people who deserve all the negative reaction cannot possibly handle it. Their bodies would become weak and their minds shattered, so the overflow must inevitably fall to the good. This theory I realize also sucks but I feel it is true.

Theory of Relative Random Probability - This theory pretty much sucks for most of us but that's the way life goes. It's an in-depth explanation of Karma. The theory states that when unordinary things happens to you, *for the worse*, it seems like random bad luck to you...but it is actually relative to who you are, what you do and what you did in the recent past. It is probable that you deserve something bad to happen to you whether you care to admit it or not. This is a relative reaction to a random negative incident that you caused before. Karma can be a powerful ally for some and it is very often disregarded.

Theory of the God's Big Bang - God doesn't care what you think created the universe. This is a two part theory. The first part is mine and I came up with the name. The second part is not mine but it is so significant that it requires printing. Part one: While God created the Earth and man in 7 days (7,000 years), we are not at the center of our galaxy or the universe as we know it so He probably created another race of "man" first and while the events of the Bible probably did happen as Genesis explains, we are likely just a younger copy of the original. Part two: God (in being all of everything) may choose what company in He wishes to keep in heaven. God has already done so by creating good souls and bad souls so that the good can learn from the mistakes of the bad in this life. After death God reclaims His chosen in Heaven and the rest go somewhere else. This sucks if you are one of the latter, but it makes sense. Some people are pre-doomed to do bad things and while other people do seemingly good deeds, if the deed does not glorify God according to the Bible, then it is not actually good. There's a big fat pill to swallow for some of you.

Theory of Named Destiny - This theory says that for the most part the name you give your child will pre-destine many aspects of their formative adolescent and adult lives. You are not condemning or gifting them, however they would have to be exceptional children in order to break the mold. It is possible though. Don't get pissy. I am including some examples so you can see that for the most part I am correct:

Name	Pre-Destiny
Rachael	Beautiful and highly intelligent but very closed off. Well adjusted internally and resourceful but also very careful. Idealistic and proud. Accomplishments mean a lot.
Erin (girl)	Very intelligent and absolutely stunning! When born under the right signs they have an intense physical magnetism about them. They carry themselves well and will have great reputations. Prone to rash decision making and over-reacting. The last one I met broke my heart.
Stephanie	Always popular girls and usually pretty but bad judges of character when it comes to choosing the right man. Naturally the center of attention.
Robert/ Bob	Always a well adjusted boy or man. Very dedicated and loyal. Humorous. Often times extremely intelligent and borderline OCD. They can be cunning but faithful.
Lori	Tendencies toward sexual over activeness at early ages regardless of body type. Deviant. Emotionally unstable, irrational, and eventually borderline if not fully psychotic.

Jason	Angry and sometimes violent. Socially unskilled and bad at communication with others. Cannot accurately express feelings. Smart enough to get ahead but often arrogant.
Gary	Prone to gayness and early hair loss. A high percentage will be involved with math or engineering. Almost no personality before age 50.

Now these are frequently correct assumptions but they are not the rule. Don't get all pissy. We all have faults.

**I did know a girl named Lori from High School who was extremely smart and a fox as well. She was neither psychotic nor overactive. I had nothing but respect for her and to my knowledge she turned out well. I have also been slapped by several unstable Lori's. It should be noted that I never put it in the back door either so it was totally unjustified.

If your name is one that I have listed above and you do not fit one of the negative descriptions then consider yourself a lucky person who had good parents. If you do fit the description then you should realize that the whole world has now been given the ability to see what an ass you really are. Please change your ways and try to become a better person.

ALL THINGS DRINKING

OK, so I bet this is what you were looking for from several chapters ago! Information and rules on the Heavy Drinkers Club; "Association" would have sounded better but we were drunk. When I started drinking I actually had a goal in mind. I wanted to be a professional. If I was going to do it I wanted to be able to do it right and not choke in front of everybody at the bar. All of the old cowboys who walked into the bar and slammed several shots of whisky seemed like pretty tough, cool guys so that was it. I wanted to be able to take shots like a man of the old west who was really upset about his whole life and somebody stole his horse and shot his dog. Nowadays I drink so I can tolerate society.

Here's one that not everybody can stomach, literally. The good old Heavy Drinkers Club. Just drinking on your own is fine I guess but drinking with a goal in mind is better. Don't you like the way that the guys in the movies are always able to take shots without ever flinching. That was my reason for joining up and at one point I could do it too but that doesn't last for the rest of your life. It's a limited engagement. I stopped drinking to the point of getting stupid right after college. It just wasn't as much fun anymore.

The initiation I took was as follows but I'm sure there are variations on the matter:

> -One full really nasty beer in a can like
> "Dog Style or Old Milwaukee's Beast"

> -One shot of the Three Wise Men
> Jim Beam / Jack Daniels / Jose Cuervo

> -One more full really nasty beer in a can

> -One shot of Wild Turkey to represent the beast in us all.

> -One final full really nasty beer in a can

The really nasty beer **has to be** the nastiest that you can find so that it's hard to take down quickly and burns like acid. If it's got dirt in it; all the better. You drank all of that as quickly as possible. The key is, that was just the first round. You still have to drink more beer for several hours and do shots of car bombs and _cement mixers_ (these are sooo nasty) AND then still eat barbecue food and spaghetti. (There was a great all-niter in downtown Omaha for this called The Smoke Pit). One more thing, you had to keep it all down until after you got home at 3am and went to bed. That's where the masses will fail, but don't feel bad. If you projectile vomit in the morning, you're still in. You just can't projectile vomit before you go to bed. In fact I don't even recommend you try this.

Once you are in then you are free to experiment with all manner and variety of shots without the fear of ever being labeled as a puss in public. You don't ever have to drink that hard again, but you proved (in front of at least three witnesses) that you could.

Below are some good old-fashioned drinks which I find to be personally awakening, two of which (the Creamy Smurf and the Underground River) I created all by myself way back somewhere about 1988 or so. You are welcome to the recipes. All of these are on my regular list. I do not claim to even know where some of them came from. I write these things on scrap pieces of paper when I am drunk and possibly not even in the country, so I am therefore excused from notations in this section by citing International Maritime Law. In short it states: If you are in international waters and drunk at the same time you are clearly not responsible for the content of any material you might write on a napkin.

You will notice that most recipes do not contain measurements. That is because unless you are baking at high altitudes or pouring oil into a car, measurements are for pussies! Just mix it until it tastes good. If you get a little too much booze and you still drink it, you are a better person for having done so. Enjoy.

Creamy Smurf	Medium Juice Glass. Blueberry schnapps / Blue Curacao / Irish Cream and a cherry or other red fruit for the Smurfberry.
Underground River	Splash of Orange Juice for bottom layer / small shot Blue Curacao middle layer / equal size shot Brandy on top / cherry garnish
Jamaican 10-speed	Midori / Malibu Rum / Banana Liqueur / 4 parts Cream / 4 parts Pineapple Juice / Lime garnish
White Russian	Vodka / Kahlua / Milk or Cream Served over ice because milk will separate
Manhattan	Whisky / Sweet or Dry Vermouth / Angostura Bitters / Cherry garnish
High ball	Ginger ale / Whisky
Champs Elysses	Grenadine / Cognac Brown Cream de Cacao Orange Curacao Green Cream de Menthe
Screaming Orgasm	Irish cream / Kahlua / Vodka / Amaretto
Kamikaze	Mostly Vodka / Cointreau / Rose's Lime
Cement Mixer	Irish Cream / Rose's Lime. Swish around in mouth until the ingredients coagulate like Jell-O and then attempt to swallow.

Mai-tai	1oz rum (or 151 rum) / ½ oz orange Curacao / ½ oz Rose's Lime / almond syrup / Lime Juice and Cherry
Tequila sunrise	tequila / ½ oz grenadine / Orange Juice / Cherry
Bar Swill	You get a tray & have the bartender pour all the drinks over that for ½ hour. You get what you get & it's pretty nasty.
Fuzzy Navel	O.J. / Peach Schnapps / and mine come with Apricot Brandy for extra fuzziness.
Cherry Bomb	½ oz Cherry Brandy / 1oz Rum / ½ oz Sour Mix

<u>Honorable mention</u>

The Margarita	If you have to have more than 1 then you didn't make it right. The original was made in 1948 I believe with Grand Marnier so insist on that & real lime juice, no pre-mix crap. Real agave nectar is totally acceptable w/ lime juice. Add a floater of Frangelico to make it really awesome.

If I had anything else to say on the subject it would be this; Go and perform all of your Christmas shopping while you are absolutely blasted. It will make you laugh. People at the mall are great entertainment especially when you are in this state. Your gift recipients will never ask for anything from you again and it takes the stress out of that season. It's really not about shopping anyway so why not go ahead and fuck it up real good for everyone who thinks it is? That sounds like a good bit of logic to me. I personally have been doing this for over 10 years now and I am very satisfied with the results. Remember, Christ's birth day is actually in September anyway. Look to the Jewish calendar to verify that it's true. December should just be called "Cold Weather Drinking and Sex Month". Thank you.

TRAINS

Now no one can deny the fact that smashing things into oblivion is cool. Destruction is very cool! Explosions are great. Being as how I like to watch these sorts of things, it was an important part of my college career to get a friend, get some beers or other hard liquor and go find some stuff to put on the tracks. Yes 95% of the time we were drunk but that made the explosions and combustions seem better and the trains were louder, faster and bigger. Sometimes we would even put a recliner (for example) on the tracks and then situate ourselves down by tracks under a bridge or on top of another. My dear friend Michael had a pension for peeing on the train as it went by. I never really got into it although I probably did pee on one or two.

It should be noted that doing anything on railroad tracks including walking on them for any distance is against the law. Smashing things is even more against the law, so just beware.

The point is that smashing things amuses people and it always has. Demolition Derbys have attracted people for a good long time and I think that the ante should be raised now to include locomotives. Have you ever seen a train plow through a chest of drawers? It's a beautiful thing! We could go large scale with it though and include letting children watch tank/train hybrids plow through ghetto houses that are all boarded up. They make our streets look nasty anyway and it will encourage the neighbors not to let their houses degrade and our children will want to keep things nice.

Trains can also be used for good things like shipping bums and criminals to Iowa. They may produce food there, but that is one gay-ass lame-o state if I have ever seen one. It's boring and should be converted into a large penitentiary or nuked into the ground and filled to become another great lake. Trains and cars should be allowed to go extra fast there. Why do we not have bullet trains in the U.S. anyway? Did we just decide that we didn't need anything that fast? Japan is a tiny little country and they use them. I want to go 300+ mph damn it!

NUDIE BARS

Nudie bars are not all bad. Many of them could stand to be cleaner establishments and not brick shanties on the outside but the concept is good though. There is nothing wrong with paying to see people get naked. At some time in your adult life you will try to imagine (if you want to or not) at least 60% of the people you meet in that way. For some of us it's a lot more, admittedly. I think we should have family nights at the nudie bars as a method of social gathering between married couples and families with children. Let the kids get a free feel of some things so they know what's going on out there.

The people who "dance" have to break down and admit one thing though. Unless you live by the book and work in a really nice cabaret or dance hall; you are a whore. As long as you can admit that to everyone you meet then I don't have a problem with it. There are some times in the lives of millions of people that call for a good whore. It can be a man-whore too. The rules apply to both sides. The odds of you not being a whore are simply astronomical so let's not talk about it further.

One thing we can do to knock down the whore stereotype is to discourage the practice of giving money directly to the dancers on a stage. It's kind of belittling anyway I tend to think. Tip at the door on the way out and give 'em some applause for working hard. I don't like tipping anyone in person. It just seems wrong and it shouldn't be an expectation. One day I am going to tip dancers with Oreo™ Cookies under the strap. Oreo pasties would be totally hot!

Shouldn't they have intermissions at the bar like in a hockey game when the Zamboni comes out? They could run a 10 minute cartoon projected on the wall while they re-wax the poles and decontaminate the floors.

2012 END OF DAYS?

I am personally, *absolutely fascinated* with this shit. Its crazy what's going on there and how it all seems to be connected and pointing to our downfall. This could be a whole chapter by itself but I am trying to show self restraint.

There are supposedly huge bunkers and arks in Russia and Norway. I have heard some things about scrolls uncovered in Iraq that could cause destruction and they were the secret cause for the whole war. I have heard that the aliens are fully aware of the 2012 timeline. Are they a part of the impending disaster or merely observing it? Will they save anyone? Now I even hear that President Obama was supposed to have announced their legitimate presence around Earth on television. We have had meetings with several races and supposedly the governments of the world agree that it would be a better idea to wait for disclosure until after the population has been drastically thinned out. What does that mean? If it is true, it tells me that they all agree on disaster in 2012. Leaders are not likely to tell us what they are doing now to prepare since we have a shitty economy. Any of this stuff would certainly make a lot of people freak out and panic though. That would cause some end of the world style shit to start falling mainly because it would directly conflict with the greater populations' limited view of God and the universe.

People have also asked me to compare my notes to those of the popular *FICTION* series Left Behind that has in fact sold 15+million copies or so. It's good. I read it and I liked it. It has its basis in biblical references, but its still fiction all the way up until it actually happens. That is the distinguishing point. It is written in the future tense.

You do also have the anti-Christ / religious angle. This is a person of flesh, not the devil himself. Going forward this is important for you to distinguish. So you have the book of Revelations and similar texts from other religions. They pretty distinctly describe events that will take place in the future that will indicate the end of world (as we know it) may be upon us. Some say that Revelations directly refers to star charts and astrological events. Do an internet search on Daniel's Timeline to find out more. It basically matches up these star charts with both the Lunar and the Gregorian calendars to give us a shit falling from the sky start date of _evening - March 21st 2013_ (not that far off from Dec. 2012) and also a date for Jesus' return to earth of pretty much _September 2nd 2016;_ then it all ends officially 45 days later. You have to look at it for yourselves. I could easily buy into it.

The Mayan calendar ends on 12/21/2012, and Nostradamus predicted that man would have a choice to live in peace or destroy each other at that time as well (nearing 2012). We also know that all the shit will fall apart in the Middle East and Israel will be the center of the battleground. When it became a recognized nation again some 50 years ago, people got worried instantly, but the other pieces of the puzzle weren't in place yet. Now that gays can get married in Iowa, that's pretty much all we needed to end it.

My point of order for every single one of you and especially our current President Obama is this; unless you unwittingly wish to become the anti-Christ, you need to stay the fück out of Israel. Things do not look good for you in this matter anyway with the whole 2012 thing I just mentioned and all of the Biblical cross connections that may be happening. It will be the end of your 1st term. Things are already going downhill over there. The anti-Christ will be a charismatic person (which you are) who makes an honest mistake before realizing it is too late and then will take the side of evil. The shit is going to go down in Israel, so just keep us out of there and you don't have to worry. Pretty simple.

As for the rest of the 2012 thing, there are multiple scenarios. I have decided that I don't believe any of the mass destruction will happen. I already own land with a cave and natural running water up in the mountains so I probably will hang out up there just in case. Really though if it did go down like that I wouldn't want to be alive for very long afterwards because life will be hard. I don't want a hard life. I like an easy life very much. I would still like to die fast, so maybe a large secondary fireball could hit me. Drowning sucks though so I'm not down for that (hence the mountains).

I did find it pretty cool that the portrayals of potential natural disasters have been pretty damn close to accurate. If it was a natural thing it would almost certainly have to start with a solar flare, which is scheduled to happen. When Al Gore's wax skin costume melts off and he is revealed as an alien then you'll know it has begun. There is also a chance that if it was bad the earth could change axis, rotation or both so that's going to screw up some plans. I need to figure out where the coast line will be in the future.

The primary thing that is never addressed though is human chaos. Even if we do get some but not all natural disasters there remains the fact that retards will be looting stores for televisions that won't work without the power grid. There also won't be any cell phone usage because they won't work with massive electro-static interruptions, so that means there will be governmental chaos as well. Furthermore your brand new fucking Lexus probably won't work because the computer chip will be too fried to allow it to start. MAYBE old cars will run...maybe. Don't try to argue with me about this point. I don't care about your feelings and opinions or how many of your fat children will burn in the fire. We're all gonna return to God someday so you best get mentally prepared for it now. I will be nice to you and your kids in heaven, I promise. You know, just for kicks if it does start to go bad, I might just light a Wal-Mart™ on fire for my own personal satisfaction. :)

When most people think of the Rapture, they think of the good people being taken to heaven, but the Bible doesn't say that exactly. It says that the chosen will be taken out of the way (after the righteous dead have been raised). I am still confused about the dead being raised part I admit, but we can't worry about that. Hopefully they will get their youthful good looks back if they stay on earth. I would rather not live with zombies as you already know. But for the living example; Noah was taken out of the way and the rest of humanity destroyed. Lot was spared when the city of Sodom was destroyed. There are more examples. I think we as Christians may have it backwards. If that is the case and the good people are spared, I don't think we'll have any clue what to do next. Just think about it.

I do hope if I am around that I can figure out a way to watch the insanity from a tower with a giant telescope. I like it when the police have to use mustard gas on the crowds. That's awesome.

...AND WHEN I'M DEAD, DEAD and GONE

I am most concerned about the way people will think of me after my body has passed on if I don't die in 2012. What legacy if any will I have left for children to awe at and learn from? What legends will I have created for others to pass on or use as an example? That's actually a big part of the reason for writing this book at all. Everybody has one inside but how many do you know that put it down? I have to be remembered for something even if it is for being an old strange man or for never fitting into the mold. I'm already known for being a creepy perv' so I might as well continue.

This whole thing comes to mind every time I see a homeless person making their way up an otherwise bustling street at a crawls pace. They have been stripped of everything and are now so void of life that now this is as fast as they can go. My friend has a very lethargic cat named Wagon. We have an understanding. We leave each other alone and respect our boundaries. In fact it only comes to me when it can't get out itself or when no one else has fed it. The point is that an animals' life cannot be that exciting. If they knew how to talk, most of them would probably be in therapy because they went stir crazy within the first year of their lives. Even they have more life than the person inching up the street. For this I have to leave something.

Now because most people don't pay attention unless you beat something into their minds, it is better to write things down so that at least when the time comes they will have a point of reference. For this reason I am now writing what I would like to look down from the spiritual plane and see at my funeral. My friend Vivian wants a party in the street with loud music and people bawling and carrying on; kind of like Mardi gras. I will do this for her.

I want an all day and all night celebration with a concert and fireworks at the end. Everyone I know should attend and if they don't I will know what a piece of crap they really are. Old friends who don't fly in from out of town will also be considered pieces of crap so if you are one and you're reading this you better come. Everyone should be made to eat only the kinds of foods I liked for the entire day including my Mashed Potato Surprise. All of my favorite music should be played including my own album if I ever get it recorded. I would also like something with a good Cuban beat at lunchtime. There should be a full service bar that is free for those who _need_ it. Every member of my family should get behind the microphone (even the shy ones) and say what they felt about me good or bad. Oh this is very important too. Everyone should wear bright primary and secondary colors. Not together in a rainbow though because God says "Don't be gay; Please obey". Hawaiian shirts are totally acceptable with sandals and no pants.

This event should be held on a warm beach somewhere, so if I die in the winter then you'll have to preserve me for a while or go to the equator. There should be young girls in bikinis dancing with the old men. I don't care, pay them if you have to but I want to see young flesh. I want the memory of this party to be forever burned into the minds of those who came so that when they think of it they will tell stories of me and the time I gave them.

What I would like to have done with my body is a hard call for me. I know that I would like to have a mausoleum built instead of just a gravestone. It should be big enough for people to walk into but also be well lit with windows. A healthy bit of quartz would be nice mixed in with the cement marble and granite. Held within these walls should be some of my most prized possessions like Transformers, microphones, my instruments, and of course a laminated copy of my works also burned onto CD.

I think that I would like to be cremated in the fashion that Darth Vader was burned in the "Return of the Jedi" on a tall wooden edifice so that my ashes and spirit can go up into the sky. It is my goal to own beach property somewhere so then my ashes should first be mixed with those of my beloved puppy Daisy and then dispersed onto the beach. Mix them in with the sand and mark the area as sacred ground. Do not cover the ground with anything though and we should not be bound in any container. Our souls will be happy and free.

In my mausoleum, which is just the physical place of remembrance (well removed from the burial site) should be a nice collage or presentation of pictures of Daisy and I.

A mausoleum might be nice. We don't build those anymore.

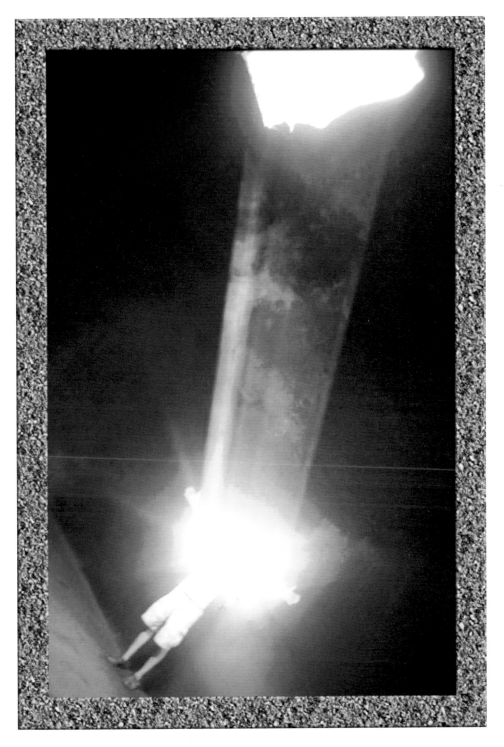

DO YOU SEE THE LIGHT?

From arguably the greatest movie of all time this title comes from the Blues Brothers movie so you have to say it in your mind like James Brown: _"The jingle-jangle of 1,000 lost souls?"_ Preach it brother! I want to go to the Triple Rock Baptist Church. I love that music. I love New Orleans style pipe worship. Flying brown people, ABSOLUTELY!

Yes! Yes! Jesus H tap dancing Christ I have seen the light!

This picture was taken on filming location for the Giant Monster Movie "Sacrifice". No special effects were added to this picture. There wasn't too much I could do in the way of turning it since I am not a Photoshop master. My niece just took this as I stood in the ray of light coming through a hole in the top of the building. We made this look like a cave and so we had thrown dirt everywhere. It was just beginning to settle at the right time. I think it was about 9:30am in Cave Creek, AZ. You would think that I was wearing a shiny shirt or a mirror necklace, but nope. It is just the light of my brilliance coming off a (dirty) white HANES t-shirt.

That is a brilliant light but it's said that you cannot even look at God while you are alive. Your body would be vaporized. Moses asked God if he could see him and was told "no, you cannot" so that's pretty cool.

Photographer: Aura N.

SPIRITUALLY MEDICATED

CHAPTER XIII

We had to move this to the back 'cause its more informational and boring than the rest of the book. I felt it a necessary inclusion though because most of you are so ignorant. It is still a slap in the face, just not as hard.

I am far, far, far from being a biblical reference. I am not ashamed to say that I had to look some of this stuff up. I knew it was in there because I do have a solid foundation, but that's why we have religious books, right? So we can look stuff up for ourselves.

This chapter wasn't supposed to be that long because there were spiritual undertones all through the rest of the book. It turned ugly on me the moment I decided to compare the different religions. I want you to consult an authority on the subject should you become more interested.

I will tell you that I had a strong religious upbringing and although I believed, I drifted away for a long time. You are learning my story now. I like many of you have personal struggles. Returning home to God has changed my life. It's not perfect and my cup of tolerance is still rather shallow but comparatively to just drinking all the time and living with lots of hatred at least I see the light!

So you need to fix your life. Don't ignore your problems. I should have taken my wife to church. I should have gone more myself. When I finally came back in the literal sense of walking through the sanctuary doors I was hesitant. You have to first let go of the notion that God isn't real and that church won't do anything for you. That is a defeatist attitude that you need to get rid of. If you carry that inside, of course it's not going to work for you. Literally billions of people can't be 100% wrong. There's got to be more.

FORMAL RELIGION

Formal religion is bad at all. It's just not for a lot of people. Christianity as a formal world religion was developed by the Roman government and used as a method of controlling its' citizens. Constantine was the Roman ruler credited with the creation of a council that would decide on the current books of the bible; what was to be changed and what was to be omitted. This is a point of contention for many non church goers. Truly this is just an excuse not to seek God as one should. I find that the individuals who like to play that card when confronted are often misguided about the very subject. You can still find those writings! Many of them are in what is called an Apocrypha. There are also many ancient texts still around from which we can derive the truth about the books before this instance occurred. It's not like we really lost this information.

What's really funny to me is that the participants of every religion constantly demean the other global religions. You fools are all worshiping the same God. You just speak different languages and let your cultural differences get in the way. We are great fighters amongst ourselves. I have witnessed some ugly church dealings take place apart from the ordinary denominational things between Baptist, Methodist, Lutheran, Protestant, etc... I saw a worship arts pastor be fired for inspiring people to worship too much. Figure that one out. The congregation was told it was actually a worship style conflict with the lead pastor although a bit of it was interpersonal I'm sure. You just don't fire a great musician for playing too well.

Despite all of our eternal bickering I will attempt to show you how it is that we created sects amongst ourselves and from where we all came. The ties that link us all are quite interesting.

I believe in God.

I believe that many spiritual leaders from all across the globe existed and some performed miracles. I believe in Jesus as the enlightened Son of God, but I am a Son of God as well. I believe in the teachings of Buddha and I might believe in Vishnu as well, had I read the Hindu scriptures, but they all refer to the same creator of the universe so I fail to see the point other than to be diverse and accepting. I write about this in the alien chapter as well because they believe in the same God! It's good stuff.

I think that some form of religion, even if you have created your own way to worship, is good for everyone. It has its place and it serves to help us all be kinder gentler beings. But you must take a more active role in your own life and start being responsible for your own actions. God, Jesus and the Holy Spirit do love you unconditionally but I don't believe that they approve of all the nonsense that takes place here on earth.

BEING ONE WITH THE PEW

"If you're gonna go to church, do some churchin'!" *Churchin'* in that sentence is being used as a Deep South verb. It means don't bother to go and just be a wallflower. You're supposed to worship God so get to it. The church is your safe place. If you can't feel comfortable raising your hands up to God and singing within those walls, then you probably need to re-evaluate your life and why you are there. Eventually you will come back to square as the saying goes. You might have 80 years behind you before you feel like you can release yourself and start to worship. As long as you get there my friends, that's the important thing.

The topic of God and spirituality is something that nobody likes to talk about. They will, but they have to be goaded into the conversation. We don't do a nearly good enough job as Christians in regards to behaving like friends and leaders. If we did, it would be easy to go out on the streets and find someone instantly with whom you could comfortably talk about God. There are some people out there that do proclaim it in their daily lives, but not the majority of us.

In early 2009 I watched Kurt Warner first and foremost publically give thanks to Jesus after the AZ Cardinals finally made it to the Super Bowl. That for me was a cool thing to witness. Whatever name you choose, it is more than ok to be a witness or give testimony in public. We all worship the same living God.

TITHING

I am going to hit this hard and fast, directly after formal religion since that's where it fits. If you like your place of worship, which you should, then it is absolutely essential to tithe. I have one and only one problem with where the money goes. The act of tithing is primarily to help the impoverished people through the church. It is not an intended mechanism for anyone to be wealthy. No Pastor, Bishop, Rabbi or anyone of the sort deserves to make as a salary one hay-penny more than $100,000. I'll say this later in another chapter just for emphasis. It doesn't even matter how charismatic you are or how many lives you touch with your inspirational message. How can you even stand up and preach to people about hardship? It doesn't even matter how many children you have made or adopted. If you accept a paycheck larger than that, you then are a hypocrite. Take some time off and figure it out for yourself.

PROFANITY and HYPOCRISY

I feel like I have to say this over and over again. Because of the nature of this book, you have to have an open mind. I swear that if I am doing a book signing and a fanatic comes up to me and wants to argue about anything, I will personally beat your ass in the book store. Yes, I am also heavily armed at all times. People who have a closed mind really annoy the lukewarm piss out of me and that is one of my huge T.S. triggers.

I have to address the issue of my profanity as it relates to God early on in this book; otherwise I will come under even more scrutiny than I already anticipate. God does not want us to have filthy mouths or filthy minds. This is a general rule. God _commanded_ that we not take His name in vain. So if you have to swear, do your best to not swear _against_ God. My Mother explained this to me when I asked her about it at age 12. I was literally afraid of death by lightning if I cursed. I'm not joking! So she explained; "When a person says God Damn It, they are literally asking the Lord to send something or someone into damnation. Be careful not to say that about another person, but if you stub your toe on the bed and you want God to damn the bed frame then that's ok. Just know what you're saying." Again, my Mother the Sage...

One of the things that people feel obligated to say to me is "How can I call myself a Christian when outward appearances lean to the contrary". I do not dispute that I can come across as an asshole. What I will dispute all day long is the fact that I am one of the kindest most God-fearing men that I know. You can assume that I am not perfect and you would be right, but I try. For all the challenges that arise in life I am proud to say that I do a good job. In the words of one of my pastors "It is more important to run a good race through the course of your life and to finish strong than it is to have fleeting moments of strength."

I am also proud to say that much of the relief that I have found has come from a rich church centered life and a devotion to God. It just makes me happy.

CREATION

Everybody loves to ask me my views about the creation of Earth because they know they will get an honest answer from me and maybe even one they hadn't thought of yet. The subject seems rather simple and not something that I would consider an issue at all, however much like in politics there seems to be only 2 camps. Either you believe in biblical creation or you believe in a bang theory leading to evolution. I am here to say that if you can't open your eyes to the following philosophy then you are indeed blind.

If you look around you and inside yourself and you don't believe that a higher being had a hand in your creation and in that of the wonders of the planet that you are on, then you my square-headed friend are not worthy of the salt and water that you are made from. Truly, truly I say to you that none of us is worthy anyway, but the Lord has placed each of us accordingly and with full knowledge of our short comings He allows us to live by his grace alone. I dally, so let's continue.

The biblical camp claims that the Earth was created in 7 days while the evolutionist camp claims that the Earth is roughly 4.5 billion years old. Don't quote me on this, it is irrelevant. If you are on team bible then by default you are saying that the Earth is roughly 30,000 years old. That's a big difference! I purpose that God does not play according to the clock of man! Just 1 of those 7 days may be equivalent to 750 million years through the eyes of God. So who are we to dispute that as a possibility?

It goes on in the same manner. One person says that God put dinosaur bones in the ground to test us and another uses those same bones as irrefutable proof of life much longer than 2 days before man came along to name the creatures. Why can't it be something in the middle? Again, God's days were long. He did make dinosaurs; thought about it for a while. They didn't really fit into the plan so well, so God creates a meteor and erases them. He gives life another few hours of his time to regenerate as he makes new creatures and then says, ok now we can have man, and maybe we'll give him a short tail for a while just to try that out. Come on people. Again with the fighting? Do you see how silly the one sided view looks to me?

Finally, I have one more poke in the side for you, and it's not even my thought. What if God created the "big bang"? I'm just rehashing for the sake of people who don't watch Anime. I know at least 3 people who watched Akira and didn't even make the connection. That or they didn't make it to the end of the movie. Ha ha.

PERSONAL STRUGGLES

"God does not owe you anything. You owe God." - Me (3/27/09 over coffee watching snow fall). That doesn't mean that He wants to see you struggle but Earth is definitely not Heaven!

We have to work here. We have to go through not _some_, but _many_ unpleasant things so that we learn and grow. Sometimes that does include cancer. Sometimes in involves foreclosure. Just deal with it. Give up all the crap in your life and get back to basics. God doesn't mind if you make money. I suspect God reserves the right to spank you with the Karma Paddle if you act like a rich jack ass though.

I just told you many of my problems, but as for what becomes of me, only God knows. Personally I know that I need to be loved really well by at least one woman (maybe 4) in order to release my gifts to others. It's not codependence. I just don't function well without a counterbalance. Every wound to my heart contributes to my inevitable fatality. I am a man of royal insistence. I must know, I must feel, I must be. <u>So where does this leave me now?</u> There sometimes seems to be nothing that I can give God in order to get an answer.

So in the interest of sharing, here are some more things that many people including myself face. These are challenges that we must help each other to overcome:

<u>Why should I go to church?</u> It certainly is not the place where everything is supposed to be perfect. Indeed it is the opposite. If you can't bring your problems to the Lord (who already knows all your troubles) then who can you turn to? Church is supposed to be the place where it is alright to cry, ask for help and bring the junk from your trunk. Fellowship is a huge part of the whole thing. Everyone needs to feel like they belong. The church can be your community and your family if you let them. The Jewish people have a wonderful dinner style gathering they call a Shabbat. It is held with your religious family and not just within your own bloodline. It is a time of reflection and study as well as social interaction and support.

<u>What should I be waiting for and for how long must I be patient?</u>
These questions just piss me off all day long. There are 2 stories that I recall about people being patient and it really didn't go so well for either of them, although they did do what was right in the eyes of God. People always say "Never ask for the patience of Job" and I do not. I just want enough to make it through the day without anxiety.

As for how long does one have to wait; well there is a story about a man who waits 7 years to marry the woman he loves, only to be tricked into marring her sister. Then he has to wait another 7 years to marry Rachael! I am not trying to be that patient. Lord, take me pretty! Take me now if I have to wait that long. It ain't worth it! I can put up with a lot from a woman when I'm with her, but to have to put in 14 years of labor before I even get the slightest hint of a reward, come on. And then you still have to work on the marriage. It's not just perfect from day 1. I'm tired and upset now just thinking about it. I know you ladies think that's funny.

<u>What if I hate all of my family?</u> We are placed into families in this life for many reasons. We are sometimes able to chose to come back to finish lessons or complete journeys. We may not always like the personalities of the siblings or the parents living in our homes. We are all there to learn from each other. This sometimes becomes uncomfortable when it includes the elder learning from the younger.

<u>I don't like organized religion.</u> In every religion prophets claim that theirs are the true people of God and they have the only road to salvation. God is vast I do not believe He would put restrictions upon man that they must only follow one path to get to Him.

AFTERLIFE

Purgatory is the name that we have given to the sort of middle ground that we believe our spirits go to before we are judged. We could have chosen a better name. It sounds like you're already damned if you're there. That's not the case nor do scholars claim to know how long a person is supposed to be in that state.

I try my best to behave in this life because I really don't like being judged and I don't to be on the losing side. I would very much like to know what my role in heaven might be, other than just worshiping God. I don't know but I give it some thought. In any case I do not fear death and I agree with the old saying "Lord, take me pretty". If you've never heard that it means "I've had close to enough here on Earth. I'm not willing to take my own life since you commanded I should not, so would you consider allowing me to die now in my sleep before it gets any worse and I become fat and crippled?"

One of the reasons I think I am afflicted with TS is because in another life I must have been pretty powerful and an asshole times 4 on top of that. It would at least explain some of my dreams.

RE-INCARNATION

Everyone has their own specific views about God, Heaven and what happens to us after we're gone from this world. Believe what you like but here is my take on the subject and I am not alone in my views. As I understand it, several million Buddhists and Hindus believe much the same.

I believe that when we each were created as an individual soul out of nothing but energy that we were given a body and that most or all us didn't even start as human. Along our lives journeys we are meant to learn an indefinite amount of lessons and that when we have learned and practiced those lessons that we can move on, hopefully to a higher form. Sometimes we go backwards and revert into animals or insects again. Some religions believe that insects are their ancestors and are held in high regard. Grasshoppers are one such example of former relative which are said to be watching over us. Don't harm them and they will bring you good luck.

At any rate, you go around and around being re-born several thousands of times until you have become a truly righteous person and attempt to live your final life causing no harm to others but rather teaching and helping. Some of the lessons along the way include being in servitude to others whether it is in your job or as an actual slave. Other lessons would include coping with being ugly or fat. This is not to say that your physical appearance cannot change or be changed by your will. It is only to say that you cannot move on until you have learned the lesson that is set before you. If you have worked diligently and are no longer that way, then you can probably check that one off. There are so many lessons to learn in the world and I am always amazed at how shallow we all are. Even if you are very smart and talented you still run the risk of being shallow.

To that end I also believe that in between the smaller lessons we all have a few lifetime achievement goals. Try to think of what it is that has plagued you your whole life thus far. What have been your short comings? What compels you? I was meant to be with one person for the rest of my days. I am supposed to love and care for that person (who I asked to be my wife), and always be exactly what and where they need me to be. My other lesson is to learn to be happy with the situations that I have been given and with being poor. I am also having to learn not to ask for favors of others and to only rely on myself and my one other person (who subsequently left me posing yet another problem). These are my lifetime lessons. If I can pull them off then maybe I won't have to come back too many more times.

"Now what happens at the end of your journey then smart-ass?" Many of you have said this to me. Well that would be heaven. Utopia isn't so much a place that you go to so much as it is an altered state of being. When we have mentally evolved ourselves or have been chosen by whichever deity you believe in not to come back and be reborn then you are in your proverbial heaven. I believe that you can still walk the earth if you want to but there are other more interesting places to visit since you no longer have to pay for plane fare. The nuisances of everyday life are no longer a factor to you such as how your car is performing. You have returned the state of a being of energy, so have fun because you've earned it. Oh yes, one other final thing. <u>You'll never be done and go to heaven if you haven't experienced life for a while as a vegetarian!</u> If you don't agree with this, then your test is to stop killing and eating living animals. Suck on that meat Popsicle!

So what about Hell? Well Sir, many mediators and the worlds' forward thinkers believe hell to be more in kind to a prison. Hell isn't so much a place you go to when you die so much as it is a place you are put by other spiritual beings who are tired of dealing with you. You could be let out of this cosmic prison after a while or you could be sent back to live as somebody's bruised-up and battered cocaine bitch. Do you see the supreme justice now? I have to believe in this type of justice because it is the only thing that allows me to continue to go out into our society.

COMPARISONS

The chapter starts to get long. Right about...now!

AGNOSTIC

A person who doesn't know and basically refuses to choose what they believe in. There may be a God. There may not be. I personally find this to be a mindless position that no one of conscience could support. One might say that they do not care about the existence of God. Such a person would be lazy and useless.

ATHEIST

A person who simply does not believe in a higher being and without being shown irrefutable physical proof they are unlikely to change their position. This position is more respectable than the Agnostic because they are at least supporting a position. Atheists in essence make a two-fold statement without saying a word. If there is no God then neither humans nor anything else can have a soul. When we die then there can be no afterlife. What I do not understand about this viewpoint is the lack of acknowledgment that something sparks our life. If we didn't have flowing blood and we were instead just a spirit form with no purpose, then it could be argued that there is no God.

BUDDHISM

"Hard is the appearance of a Buddha." His life will not be easy. Neither will it be to follow the teachings yourself.

I place this section before the other religions because of very important distinctions. Internationally, Buddhism is not considered a world religion because it does not revolve around a God. Rather it encourages betterment of the self. Buddhism does not renounce God, nor does it say much about the entity. Buddha is not God. There is a differentiation. Followers seek enlightenment and those who have attained enlightenment are given the title of Buddha. Those who follow the way of the Buddha are seeking "Nirvana". This is not a fairytale place or another spiritual world but instead a state of perfect tranquility. Loosely translated the Sanskrit word I suppose would be classified as a verb meaning "to blow off/away" or "to extinguish". The Buddha Gotama spoke of Nirvana as if it were tied to death and in fact upon his death he is said to have entered into it.

In Enlightenment and Nirvana passion and pleasure do not exist in this state. That is a common misconception. Pain only exists minimally and only momentarily on a physical level. It is disregarded. Everything that is not tranquil is released from the concern of the mind.

When most of us think of a Buddha we think of the fat man statue. Admittedly, I was confused when I first saw a skinny Buddha statue; so allow me to clarify for you in steps:

The person who is considered to have been the first Buddha and the founder of the movement was the skinny one named Siddhartha Gotama. Generally, if a person speaks of only a Buddha without a subsequent name, they are referring to the Buddha Gotama. Essentially, he was a prince who gave up everything. He was born around 450 B.C. give or take 80 years near the border of Nepal and India. That's what you need to know.

Maitreya Buddha (lots of different spellings!) is the Chinese "Future Buddha" of Abundance and Happiness who is supposed to revive the spiritual movement and bring an end to suffering. The fat Buddha represents prosperity, tolerance, generosity and good luck. These are 2 additional figures and different persons entirely than the Buddha Gotama.

There was a fat monk called the "Cloth-bag Monk" who was said to be the earthly incarnation of the Maitreya Buddha. It is suggested that he was born around 850 A.D. It is from him that the image and statues are derived. There are other stories and historical figures that overlap making it almost impossible to discern the real identity of this fellow. Look on your statue to see if he has a cloth sack on his person or specifically on his back.

Jesus who was born onto earth later was also considered by many to be a Buddha.

There are many books about Buddhism. There is a "Bible" so to speak full of teachings that is called the Dhammapada.

The central teaching is that all of life is suffering. This is why I do favor Buddhism because several parts of my body and much of my mind suffer every day. I am relatively sure that you can relate to being battered or bruised on some level. This would include your pride.

The practice of Buddhism does not allow for leeway, basically telling you that if you do not follow all of its ways; you will fail. Just like Emperor Palpatine said to Luke. You will fail. The way is rigorous. It is not bad at all. It does seem like there are many more things to remember and meditate on rather than one simple mantra like "just be a good person". Here is a list of the major THINGS that you should commit to memory and adhere to. One almost has to memorize them before you can repeat them in meditation.

The core teaching is this: ***All of life is suffering***

The Eightfold Path: (represented by the Wheel of Dharma)
1) Right View
2) Right Thought / Aspirations
3) Right Speech
4) Right Behavior / Conduct
5) Right Livelihood
6) Right Effort
7) Right Mindfulness
8) Right Concentration / Meditation

The Three Refuges -or- Three Jewels:

The Buddha	(Teacher)
The Dharma	(Rules or Laws)
The Sangha	(a collective group of monks)

The Five Precepts: (Much like the commandments)
Drinking
Lying
Stealing
Harming a living being
Misuse of the senses

One does not have to become a monk to be a Buddhist although it is generally accepted that you have little chance of attaining enlightenment if you are not.

Karma: Deed or Task

Bodhisattva: Sometimes considered a lesser companion to the Buddha or also one who has reached enlightenment but came back down as it were for the benefit of others. You see, sects exist within Buddhism as with the religions. The difference in the eyes of one sect is that a Bodhisattva cares more for the welfare of others. They consider the traditional Buddha to be "self-serving" for lack of a better term. In my view it is the nature of the movement that this person should accomplish both goals simultaneously.

Dali Lama: This is a proper Title of Office given to a leader in the Gelug school of Tibetan Buddhism. He has a birth name, which in this 14th incarnation is Tenzin Gyatso.

Amida Buddha: After his earthly death, Buddha Gotama while in the state of Nirvana accumulated an innumerable amount of additional virtues. The name Amida, which means Infinite Light and Boundless Life, now precedes the title of Buddha in reference to him.   He dwells forever in what is called a Land of Purity (The equivalent of Heaven) with many other Buddha's.

There is much more to learn about this way of life but it is time to wrap up with Buddhism and move on. I did find an excellent book that I would recommend in a hotel room in Hawaii. It is called *The Teaching of Buddha* by Bukkyō Dendō Kyōkai.

4 WORLD RELIGIONS

This part could get out of hand real fast and become real long. I am striving to give you just an overview so that you are more accurately aware of the differences as seen by people of that faith or cult. For all intents and purposes we really have 4 major world religions. They are Hindu, Islam, Judaism and Christianity. Everything else can be considered either a cult or an offshoot. It has been described that a cult is really based on one of these primary religions, but it takes the essential writings or doctrines and skews them in a way that further promotes personal gain. You really don't need a whole book on this, even though they are out there. I am going to try to summarize these for you in a page each. By the way, those who claim to be atheist just chosen not to chose a side yet. Either you are religious or you believe in scientific development.

HINDUISM

A polytheistic religion much like that of mythology: I am dreading writing about this since many people of the Hindu faith cannot adequately explain it. For all intents and purposes this is a cross-reference guide to help westerners at least know the basics. I have no problem keeping this short as I do not wish to look like a complete fool!

My understanding of their concept of God is that there is indeed a Supreme Being or Existence, called the **Brahman** but that He has pretty much a "hands-off" management style toward the creation. He split into 3 essential beings but is also multi-faceted and lives in many additional forms all at the same time. Some of the forms or lesser deities may not even be aware that they are a part of this God-head. It was once explained to me that the 3 primary divisions of the God have dominion over the past (**Brahma**), present (**Vishnu**) and future (**Shiva**) respectively. Each of those deities has many beings that serve them. Anyone of the Hindu faith may worship any of the Gods including the lesser ones. The God of the Present, Vishnu is the one who is most active in our lives and therefore receives the most worship and concentration.

Hindus may change their desire to worship one deity over another in the sense that the ultimate goal is to understand all parts of the God. It is almost essential to switch focus.

To go just a little further into it, **Brahma** is the creator of our plane of existence and the origin of everything we know. He is not widely worshiped since his role has been primarily completed but nonetheless He is as important as the other 2 in terms of being a supreme deity.

Vishnu is said to be active through Avatars. This is a proper term for one who has descended to exist with us from time to time. He has 10 avatars or forms, one of which Kalki is yet to come. Other more modern recognizable forms include Buddha, Krishna and Rama. Krishna just so you know is considered a supreme God

Shiva is the destroyer and the restorer. Restoration must come out of destruction as life is cyclical. It is proper to say that He has an active role in life even though everything has not been destroyed yet as in end times.

Other than that all you need to know to round out the basics is that they do believe in the soul (called Atman). They have many, many rituals and that people of the Hindu faith often times have established places of worship in their homes. Going to a temple is not as necessary as in other religions, again because the practice is a way of life.

Entrance into Heaven: Heaven as in Buddhism is considered to be a state of being achieved when the cycle of re-birth is broken because one has learned all of their lessons.

BIBLICAL LINEAGE

According to the Bible which is the foundation for the following 3 religions, we are all descendents of Noah. Everyone prior to Noah was wiped out by the flood so that makes the lineage of Noah a pretty good starting point.

Noah had 3 sons: **Shem, Ham** and **Japheth.**

Each of these boys lived long lives and had many sons and daughters. Many could mean a whole bunch considering Shem lived for 500 years. Obviously the clans spread out over the whole world but below are a string of primary tribes. Abraham is the most prominent direct descendent as his covenant with God established him as the father of many nations and kings. He is of Shem's bloodline.

Shem → 9 generations later → Abraham

                      Ishmael – **Arabian people**
      Abraham <
                      Isaac   – **Jewish people**

Japheth – Lineage to Asia possibly??? I don't know but I am guessing by default. They were maritime/sailing people so they could have easily spread that far. Not big trouble causers and relatively little else is mentioned about his descendents.

Ham – Canaan (Cursed by Noah into being the lowest of slaves even unto his brothers. This was punishment for Ham having possibly taking liberties with his father when he was drunk and already naked) – **Dark Brown persons**

So go figure. That's where we all come from. Take it into consideration that we all came from Noah and at one point we all had the same belief system. That's where I'm going with this. Welcome to the destination.

ISLAM

A monotheistic or one God religion founded around 610 A.D. Allah is the God of Islam. Allah is not their name for him; it is more correctly a definition. Allah is _the God_. It's hard to grasp. I am told that they believe Jesus was more of a major prophet followed by another great prophet named Muhammad (because Jesus had left for Central America according to the Mormons – later; keep reading).

Again almost all of the same Old Testament scriptures apply and they believe them. So where's the big difference?

Entrance into Heaven: by acts alone.

Muslims believe that Allah would not have created Jesus as a Son. That is blasphemous. They believe that Allah had no reason to do so and that no one can die in substitution for the sins of another. That is the biggest and most direct contradiction between Islam and Christianity. The substitution of Jesus on the cross as payment in full for our sins is our foundation. Muslims hold Jesus in a place of honor and he was favored by God or Allah as he is recognized as having performed miracles. Worship is not given to Jesus. Muhammad did not perform miracles. Muhammad sinned and needed forgiveness, though he is still called Prophet. Jesus led a life free from sin and is called Messiah. They believe he was not crucified but instead taken into heaven by God. I don't know the details but I am told that they believe Judas was the man actually crucified on the cross.

Muslims worship out of duty and are saved by their acts. Rituals such as timed prayer and pilgrimage are essential in order to be acknowledged as a faithful servant of God.

Muslims are divided by 2 primary groups: the **Sunni** – Followers of Abu Bakr (Muhammad's Father-in-Law) and the **Shi'a** –

Followers of Ali (Muhammad's cousin). The fundamental argumentative point between the groups is the leadership of the religion after Muhammad passed. Since Muhammad had no living male children at the time of his death, the religion was left without a spiritual leader or as they say, one who was capable of directly communicating with Allah.

Many westerns do not understand that in many countries there is no separation between church and state.

Muhammad abandoned as a boy and raised by his Uncle. He was illiterate and so the Quran was spoken and transcribed by someone who could write. He also ordered that all copies of this work be burned or destroyed. Muslims feel that the Bible has been corrupted and therefore the Quran takes precedent over it.

Mecca is the city where Muhammad was born. It had another name but was changed after it was taken over. I think the literal translation means "the walled city" of which there are many.

A Jewish group tried to assassinate Muhammad in the city that became known as Medina. This attempt failed and Muhammad ordered the execution of many Jews. This is the event that fostered bad blood between these 2 religions.

From the Jewish standpoint, the attempt on the life of Muhammad was justifiable because he was hording all the good chocolate for himself. Well that's what I heard...

Islam has six essential beliefs that are not at all dissimilar at all to what Christians believe. They also have Five Pillars of Faith: Confession, Prayer, Fasting, Alms and the Hajj (a pilgrimage) to the city of Mecca at least once in their lifetime. None of these things are out of the ordinary for a world religion. Islam is more strict in the enforcement of their ways and the interpretation of their sacred text than some other religions. The text can be argued to support much of their actions. One might compare it to the way Greek Orthodox greatly influences the lives of its attendees.

No one may speak ill about the prophet Muhammad lest they be subject to a penalty that according to the Quran should be death. It is supposed that Allah actually told Muhammad to include this directive in the book, however it is beneficial to the leader as opposition was not allowed from the beginning.

By the design of Muhammad the Quran is supposed to be authoritative over all other books.

There is admittedly a WHOLE LOT MORE to learn about Islam and I would encourage you to do so if not for the sake of being a knowledgeable and well rounded person.

JUDAISM

For a Christian to delve into the realm of Judaism is fascinating. The study could also go on for an entire lifetime. I simply do not understand how you could be Jewish and not believe that Jesus was the incarnate son of God. I must have the story wrong otherwise all Christians should be Jewish too right? I don't get it. Why do they virtually ignore the New Testament? These are the teachings of Jesus, who by the way was a Jew. I think this is kind of an important issue to address and pretty messed up on their part. Anyway read the following section.

There are 3 key points to remotely understanding Judaism.

1) It is all about the Torah and I mean ALL ABOUT the Torah. This is a collection of the first 5 books of the Bible: Genesis, Exodus, Leviticus, Numbers and Deuteronomy.

All of these were penned by Moses. A Rabbi might connect the number 5 everywhere in the rest of the Bible to be a reference to these 5 books. If you ask about the feeding of people with 2 loaves of bread and 5 fish, don't be surprised if he says that the fish represent the 5 books of the Torah and that the people were fed spiritually. This could be the case. I don't deny it. The 2 loaves mean something too. The faith is all very symbolic.

2) The primary concern of Jews is living a good life in the here and now. They believe in an afterlife but are less concerned with it or the details of it.

3) Jews have been persecuted since the time they were established as a separate faith not wanting to be controlled by a government. We are talking thousands of years. This plays a role in their belief structure and their actions; sometimes including the denial of Jesus as Savior.

There's more to the story that is necessary for you to understand. Avoiding persecution was a huge reason to disassociate from Jesus, but also they just didn't *RECOGNIZE* him as the savior. That is the key word and it is supported in the Bible. God reveals himself not to all peoples at the same time. This is almost impossible for me to comprehend myself. Jews of the day that did follow him may have been predominately chasing physical rewards of food or health.

So even though Jesus was right there, many Jews just didn't recognize Him As long as you don't reject the Holy Spirit or the compulsory will to do good then most Jews believe you can be saved in the second resurrection 1000 years after the second coming of the Christ.

THE HOUSE OF DAVID

According to the Bible; re-establishing and bringing back together the lost tribes of the Jews is something that must happen in order for prophecy to be fulfilled. This means that Christians and Jews need to reconcile and become as one in their worship. It doesn't mean that all of us will be a part of this movement but there will be a movement and in small groups it has begun. Because there is so much to learn from each side I suspect it will take some time to grow. Go do that Daniel's Timeline search I mentioned!

HOLIDAYS

I want to mention something that is hugely important here. There is a lunar calendar that nomads followed but there exist also a religious calendar and a civic calendar. These two are offset by approximately 3½ months. In America everyone but the Jewish generally follow the religious calendar as it pertains to holidays, however this is completely inadequate and we need to stop it. As a matter of convenience for warm and fuzzy feelings I guess, we celebrate the birth of Jesus on December 25th. In fact, the event occurred sometime in the 3rd week of what we know as September. September is also supposed to have been the month in which the world was created and the beginning of the year. Understand?

The correct holiday calendar revolves around the **7 feasts of Israel**. Technically speaking these feasts and dates are something that should be observed by all servants of God. They are not just "Jewish" holidays.

The first 4 feasts are representative of the events that occurred during the first coming of Christ. These are:

1) Passover   March
2) Unleavened Bread March
3) First Fruits   March
4) Pentecost   May

The last 3 feasts represent the second coming of Christ.

5) Trumpets   September
6) Atonement   September
7) Tabernacles   September

When speaking about the end of the world and the whole 2012 thing it is important to note that Rosh Hashanah (on or about Sept. 1st) is supposed to be the day that Jesus returns marking the feast of Trumpets. Even though the Mayans and Nostradamus predict multiple things happening in December, I personally will be taking both months completely off and hiding in the mountains with guns and my beagle. God can take us up to heaven but I'm not putting up with crazy people here on earth.

Entrance into Heaven: In the faith it is called the afterlife or Olam Ha-Ba in Hebrew. They are really not that concerned with it. This is because the afterlife is not directly detailed in the Torah. Some Jews do believe in re-incarnation and it is not discredited. Some believe that according to your works and behavior one might remain in a purgatory or place of waiting until the Messiah comes again. Another common belief is that if you were terribly bad your soul will first be tortured and then altogether destroyed after 12 months and cease to exist. Similar to Mormonism, some Jews believe that not all people will be on the same level in the afterlife.

CHRISTIANITY

I know you want me to say it and I will. I am a Christian.

We have a Trinitarian God. I choose to believe in Jesus. I also believe in a God that is supreme. We exist by the grace of God alone.

People go to church every single Sunday and don't have a clue about the religion they claim to be their own. If you don't study it, then you're not that religious. Just admit it. This is especially true for the boring sects in religion whose worship times are so mundane and monotonous that it puts you to sleep. That should never be the case! That is the first sign that your spiritual life needs a wake-up call! I know this to be true. I was Lutheran. I can recite the Nicene Creed in my sleep but I would have to write the words down myself and study them in order to tell you what I was saying!

A lot of atheists say the reason they are not Christian in particular is because they hear that Constantine and the Roman government "edited" the Bible. They quote the term with heavy conviction; however it is of little consequence to me and others who are inherently good people.   There is a belief among Christians who study the word that nothing happens outside of God's will. That would include this "edit". Really, atheists are just looking for the easy out. I am telling you that everyone believes in something. They might not want to discuss it, but they do believe in something. Be it God or be it the bang or be it a peanut butter and banana sandwich.

Here's what I love about Christianity: I worship a God that loves me. I don't have to face a certain direction to pray or do it at certain times. I am thankful for everything. My salvation by the death of Christ on the cross gives me freedom. This is something I could not live without. I need you to understand that without

God being both on my side and my judge at the same time I would not be an extremely bad person. He gives me accountability. Not the U.S. Army version that requires you to get up early and say yes sir to things you don't agree with. It's the kind that makes you realize your actions may have eternal consequence. That's enough for me man! If there is a God and I'm not God; then I'm gonna do everything in my power to not make Him angry with me.

Entrance into Heaven: by faith alone. I will add that the hands of faith and works are invariably tied. One should not in good conscience call themselves a Christian if there acts reflect the polar opposite of their faith.

THE BIG FIGHT

Before you read this and for the record I am still a devout Christian. I only have the ability to see outside boundaries.

In my opinion: only one religion can be correct and therefore the others are wrong. 3 or possibly even all 4 of our world religions are wrong. We don't know which one that is. All we can do is go with what feels right in our individual hearts. I believe that when we do die God (in whatever form God truly has) will tell us;

"YOU WERE WRONG ABOUT ME IN YOUR LIFE ON EARTH. NOW I TELL YOU WHAT IS THE TRUTH AND YOU MAY SEE ME NOW AND NOT DIE. WILL YOU ACCEPT ME AS GOD? IF NOT...IT LOOKS BAD FOR YOU FROM NOW ON."

Islamic God	Christian God
Changeable Nature	Unchanging
Unknowable	Relatable
Unable to replicate	3 in 1

Is Allah the same God as the Christian God? Most of the people on Earth do not believe so, because of the fundamental difference that Christians believe Jesus is God incarnate.

MORMONS

This gets a page. Near as I can tell, they LITERALLY believe that there are 3 specific layers or divisions in Heaven and that only the 144,000 souls mentioned in REVELATION Chapter 14 will achieve the top level. They are virtually all vying for one of those spots. Without a proper understanding of the text you might think that you should strive for that in life. You should, but the point is that the souls who are referenced there are set apart by not having to ever have struggled with the choices between wrong and right. Read it, slowly, several times over.

My Mormon friends (plural intended as I have many) explained to me that their teachings provide that those on a higher plane may communicate with those on a lower plane at their discretion or more like those on the lower plane might see the others but not understand what they are doing. It could be true.

Where I find the distinction from Christianity is that they believe that after Jesus was resurrected and ascended into heaven that He in fact decided to come back down. This time He descended back to Earth in the same way landing now in Central America. From there He proceeded to teach the Indian tribes and when He was finished (I guess) He just ascended again. I had a copy of the

Book of Mormon but it grew legs and walked off so I am not about to look this up another time.

Here's where it gets funky for me. I don't doubt that Jesus did visit Central America. *It's totally irrelevant for me.* Good for those tribes-people though! All the information I need to live a good clean life is already in the Bible. I don't need another whole entire book of scriptures that say the same things. I can't barely make it through one book! I even say "can't barely" when I write about it and that is just horrible butchery of the English language.

The final thing that doesn't make sense for me is that this kid Joseph Smith presumably received some golden tablets that an Angel of the Lord told him to go find in the back woods of Vermont or something? The Indian tribes had buried them there? He could only let like 8 or 12 other people see them too and half of them were his relatives. I don't know but it doesn't make sense. If I am Jesus, first of all I don't give Americans gold tablets. That's too close to golden sheep of calves. If I did though, I would want my tablets to be on display for everyone right? I highly, highly, highly doubt that God would contradict His own word on object worship. Yes, the Ark of the Covenant had some gold on it but the Ark was made by man from the instruction of God. Stone tablets were given as the gift to man.

If someone gave Joseph Smith gold tablets those were definitely aliens posing as God. There is even recent evidence from ancient Samaria that suggests aliens were in fact mining for gold and using slave labor. Look it up.

You guys have all but slipped in another book that is supposed to take precedent and I don't see where that is a benefit to all people. It's even called *The Book of Mormon*, which is totally exclusive from people who don't join. You can't add things to scripture. That defines a cult. Play nice and think about it.

So have fun if you are Mormon. I am sorry to have to rain on the parade like this. I am not by any means putting you down. It is your choice. You are all great people and you do a lot of good for humanity. The missions you do are a blessing to many people and we are all supposed to help. Don't get mad at me for calling you out. It has already been done several hundred times in the media. Just not as bluntly. Stick to the Bible, merge with the Jews, you'll be fine.

Entrance into Heaven: by a secret handshake with an Angel and by how much better you were in life than your neighbor. The United State of Utah also intends to open their own mint and circulate pure gold coin replicas of the Joseph Smith tablets which you will have to place under your tongue. What? ...

MYTHOLOGY

I am totally fascinated with this and I always have been since I was about 8 years old. The first movie I was ever allowed to go see with just me and a friend in the theater was _Clash of the Titans_ AND it had boobs! That is what you call a win when you are 8. So all I really want to do here is break it down for you with Greek names.

There is a lot of family tree action in and amongst the Gods since they did like to break a piece off with the finer humans of the time. You should look most of this up for yourselves because it is fun to discover. Here is a short version of the Who's who. There are 10 primordial Gods of which 2 are more noteworthy. They are Kronos (Eternal Time) and Gaia (Mother Earth).

They had 4 children together. Kronos had 2 with Rhea. They are:
Demeter   Goddess of Fertility, Grain and Harvest / ½ Sister

Hestia	Goddess of Hearth and Home / ½ Sister
Poseidon	God of the Sea and Earthquakes
Hades	God of the Underworld
Hera	Goddess of Marriage / Sister and Wife of Zeus
Zeus	King of the Gods / Sky and Thunderbolts

Zeus had a whole mess of children which include the Gods:

Ares	God of War / Lover to Aphrodite
Athena	Goddess of Wisdom
Apollo	God of the Sun, Music and Healing / Twin
Artemis	Goddess of the Hunt and the Moon / Twin
Hephaestus	God of Fire and the Forge / Father of Pandora

The 3 other Major Gods include:

Dionysus	God of Wine, Festivals and Madness
Aphrodite	Goddess of Love and Beauty / Wife of Hephaestus
Hermes	God of Flight Commerce and Travelers
	(Messenger and shows the way for the dead.)

And then; way down the line (she's still a Goddess though) comes:

Nike	Goddess of Victory

Here are some of the Roman counterparts because we have named many of our planetary bodies after them. Boob Planet has yet to be found but I remain optimistic. Maybe it is Earth?

Aurora / Eos- Goddess of the Dawn
Mercury / Hermes
Venus / Aphrodite
Mars / Ares
Jupiter / Zeus
Saturn / No Greek counterpart – God of the Seed
Neptune / Poseidon
Pluto / Hades
Vulcan / Hephaestus

RELIGION TAKE AWAY

This is the single most important thing to remember from this entire chapter so it bears repeating. We could all be WRONG! I could be wrong! Aliens could be our God in disguise and Mormons would be right -or- there might be nothing after we die. Choose whatever you like. I am sticking with my choice. It makes me happy and it makes sense to me.

When we're dead and standing in the waiting room of judgment if there is one, GOD might tell everyone from every religion on Earth,

"YOU MESSED IT UP AND NO ONE GETS IN UNLESS YOU STAND BEFORE ME AND ADMIT YOUR WRONGNESS AND APOLOGIZE TO ALL YOUR PURGATORY NEIGHBORS FOR THE SIN OF CLAIMING TO HAVE BEEN RIGHT AND DISTORTING MY WILL AND MY NAME."

You can fight with GOD but you can never win.

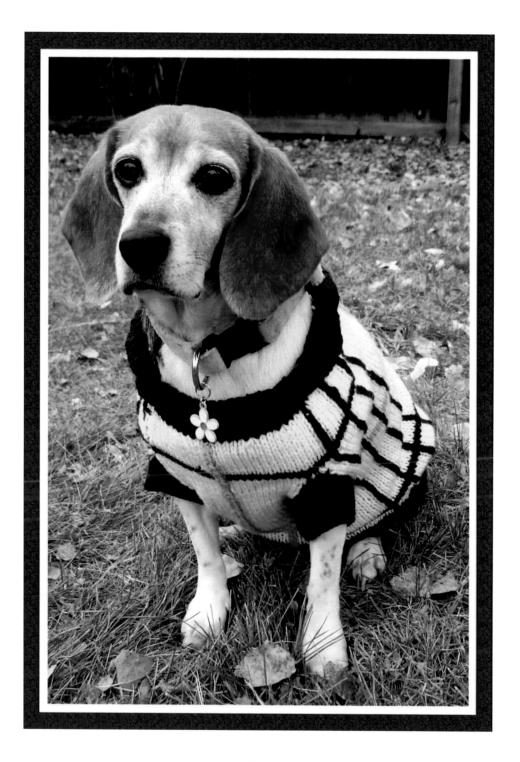

MY SHADOW

Here she is; **Daisy**. She is my love and my life. She is my inspiration. She knows roughly 35 words in English, but more importantly I know about the same in Beagleese. We make out when I come home after work and there are loud sex noises. I get to do pretty much whatever I want with her including blow raspberries on her belly. Watch our upcoming movie and you'll see. She is smarter than most human children and I guarantee she is better behaved.

Like I stated before, I have quit many projects several times. Its only when I look at her that I remember I have to carry on and finish this spite based project. We are hoping to shove this back in my ex-wife's face. If there's enough money left over I might even buy a giant billboard on a route that she drives every day. Ha ha!

This girl keeps her leprechaun magic sleeping powder in her belly and it releases when you lay down to take a nap if you put your arm under there. You're going out for 2 hours even in the middle of the day. She also has the power to make the Denver Broncos win their football games unbeknownst to them. Maybe if another team with a beach like Jacksonville wants to rename their mascot we could think about moving there.

336

IN CLOSING

THE FINAL CHAPTER XIV

I have spoken my peace. As you have seen, the bulk of my book consists of material that is designed to stir some kind of emotion in you. Most of it has been a plea of some kind to change your beliefs if they do not match mine. When people ask me if I would rather live in a world with clones of myself, I say no. What fun would that be? I only want to live in a world without hate, crime, fat, disease, or loneliness. I don't want clones necessarily but robots styled after my likeness would be cool!

I am far from perfect. I'd like to say that again. I am far from perfect, but that is my goal. I've got a lot of good years left, even though my body is pretty sore. That can be fixed with intensive massage therapy and hot water. I hope I can get there before I die so I don't have to come back again. I would like to go to the next life and have God say to me;

"YOU KNOW PAR…YOU DID SUCH A GOOD JOB LAST TIME THAT WE'VE DECIDED TO LET YOU GO BACK AS ANYTHING YOU WANT, BUT ONLY IF YOU WANT TO. WE'LL GIVE YOU SUPER POWERS, YOU CAN KEEP ALL YOUR KNOWLEDGE EVEN AS A CHILD, YOU'LL BE SURROUNDED BY LOVE AND AFFECTION, JUST PLEASE CONSIDER GOING BACK TO BE AN EXAMPLE OF WHAT AWAITS THE GOOD PEOPLE."

That's what I dream of. Frankly, I don't want to come back though. God Himself would have to personally send me back otherwise I'm done.

Maybe if you would all stop disappointing me then it would be different. We'll see. You know, I do hope that I find the next love of my life before this goes to print and she is able to stick with me through it all. That is the kind of love that renews faith.

My other goal is to get rid of all the physical things that I own so they can't continue to tether me down to one place or cause me grief if they get destroyed in a fire. I'm 40. I had to stop caring about "stuff" last year when we determined it was causing me daily anxiety. It was a shame too because I really had some awesome original Transformers™ and Star Wars™ toys.

AS MY BOOK ENDS

This is the recipe for "How to make 2 lovers of friends":

The old song title is *I Could Write a Book* with lyrics by Lorenz Hart and music by Richard Rodgers. Written in 1940 for the Musical *"Pal Joey";* we were blessed with a great recording by the voice of Ella Fitzgerald in 1959. There have been many others:

> If they asked me, I could write a book.
> About the way you walk and whisper and look.
> I could write a preface on how we met,
> So the world would never forget.
> And the simple secret of the plot
> Is just to tell them that I love you, a lot.
> And the world discovers as my book ends,
> How to make two lovers of friends.

So how many licks does it take to get to the center of a... oh, wrong question. What does it take to make 2 lovers of friends? The simple answer is "Get in bed and do it." That makes you lovers by default of having done each other. It shouldn't be a problem. Only young people confuse sex with love.

I understand that the meaning behind the verse is "How do you make lifetime lovers and marriage partners out of friends". To that I really had hoped I would be able to tell you. I failed. I tried and I gave it my all but the love wasn't reciprocal. It could have been and should have been. Here's the important lesson. _Don't over-analyze your feelings for someone until they die away._ Do something about them and live without regrets. I imagine it takes these other things as well which I did give.

Time: The kind of time that a person speaks of when they become involved with a stranger and they say, "I think we should be best friends". Well that takes maybe years; and then how much more time does it take for you to get over your fears and take the next step? It is sometimes out of your hands, but know this; it only takes one second to realize that you have been in love the whole time and you screwed it up. So what is stopping you?

Trust: Unconditional trust. I know you have my best interests at heart. I know you would lay down your life for me and/or my child. I know beyond all doubt that you act correctly because I hold a part of you and when we are not together it pains you in every moment. You are not the same without me and there is value to that loss.

This is my scripture for potential lovers:

"Too many people hold back their love from the person who truly deserves it the most. Take the chance! It's already on the table. You know you care greatly about each other. I have to love you because we were made to be together before we were born. Time would bring us together if we were 30 or 60. When I'm 60 sweetheart my stuff won't be as good! Let us not burn another moment of our bliss that the Lord God has intended. This life is short and I want to know you and love you in the next life as well. There is an act of love that we can commit. It is good. Be my lover in body and soul and we will live together in peace till the end our days and beyond."

I am sad to say that it has not worked that way for me. Let's face it, I have some real problems. Nothing insurmountable but I seem to require the attention of a lover first. I can be your friend with much more ease. For those loses I am just a little bit sad.

CREDITS and COMMUNICATIONS

This book is filled with many opinions. Please feel free to comment on all of them, as you like. Please feel free to send me email expressing your opinions as well. You can also address your concerns to my publishing company so they know that the book has impacted your life, and I will pick them up. I cannot possibly respond to everyone, and more than likely since I am lazy and take naps I won't try to do many, but rest assured that if you took the time to write down your feelings as I did then I will read them! I really only want to hear your good stories about a change you made in your life or requests to be a PAID consultant / guest speaker.

www.dpmedia.org

Don't ask me open-ended, loaded or leading questions. I hate them and I think they are a giant waste of time. You're not likely to get the response you want out of me. People have tried it for years and I know what to listen for, so I'll just fuck with you instead. Please do not send any threatening mail. It is unnecessary and uncouth. Besides, you won't be able to find me. I am cashing out and leaving the country!

It is very important to me that I give great thanks, gratitude and appreciation to those people in my life who have not only touched me but also made me whole. Among these are truly the most wonderful and loving parents a being could hope to receive; those would be mine Doug and Sharon. I would also like to include the host of my gracious relatives including my beautiful Aunt Di who put every faith in my abilities and convictions. My brothers, Tate and Shane who let me help mold them without their knowledge.

To my best friend Admiral Bob Nelson who has worked harder than I ever could, I suppose I owe you a steak dinner. He commands respect from anyone who appreciates the nuances of life. He is someone who has always been there for me and likewise. A free spirit and a man like no other and I thank him for his dedication and devotion to himself, his wife Sharon and my 3 loving nieces Zoe, Harmony and Aura. Uncle P loves you all.

My dear friend *Viviana* is truly a beautiful person. She is the Bodhisattva of Truth. So rare is she that I am fortunate to be one of the few people who can understand and feel the need for joy in her soul. She is the missing jewel in a crown and she is proud to be better than the rest, which she is. I could only ever give you love and laughter.

Carissa was a person in my life that did not have an easy time being my friend and wife. She unwittingly inspired me to be a more honest, courageous, respectful and loving person. Her support and love was unquestionable for years. I wrote this entire book either before or after our marriage but outside of our

341

time together and had hoped it would be finished while we still were. I am sorry I did not help you more. While we were married I had nothing but good things to say about most of life. Indeed, I did put off writing and several other hobbies for a while because I was that content. I hope you can change and be a good person again. Good luck.

Now I have to go with just a few first names here to protect people but also let them know what they mean to me:

- My 1st love Kimberly. I really do not know what happened or why it is that you seem to hate me. If there is something to apologize for, then please accept mine. You may call me anytime.

- My little blond friend-girl from Nebraska who asked to remain completely nameless but who helped me to grow when I didn't want to. You actually helped to stir my faith!

- Trevor, you are actually a stud and even though I am more cool, I will always have a seed of jealousy for you my friend!

- My closest and sweet young adult friend Tammy, with whom I rarely speak anymore, but who I feel I am always with. We helped each other through some interesting trials.

- My dearest friend Joan and who deserves all the best the world can give her. You know what love is and I pray that you will come to have it again with a partner. Allow yourself what you have what is good and right.

- Matt and Katie, may you never get divorced. You better learn my lessons. I love you both. We're family. I may have to hide in your house someday.

- *Cariña*, you are just the sweetest thing ever. Please stay close to me. I need you. We're a mess made in heaven.

These are people who have melted my heart in record time. I have told you who you are and as my friends you can come stay with Daisy and I anytime!

<u>Most of all</u> is my truest love Daisy. Even though she is a Beagle, she is truly the light of my Earth-bound life. She is everything I have never found in a human woman and more. I love the bellowing way she greets me when I come home and how she looks at me in the morning. I spend my free moments thinking about her when she is not with me. Most importantly, I love the way that she saved me at a time when I was about to leave the country and start a life as a bartender in Spain. (Not that we might not still make it there) I had just about enough of trying with life when my little angel came to me. We share the same birthday and she came home and slept on Daddy's chest at 5 weeks old!

To everyone else with whom I have ever shared a conversation, a drink or a laugh; I thank you too. One day I think it would be delightful to have a drink with the Muppets™ Fozzy Bear and Sam the Eagle. The complete lack of respect they share for each other and the dichotomy of their personalities would inevitably make it the most uncomfortable yet entertaining of moments.

That's all I've got. I wake up in the middle of the night and scribble things on paper. This is what is found when I thought life was getting tough one time;

"I try but I'm a tired, cranky old man and the world has gotten the better of me." –Author 12/31/07

LAST CALL

Obviously being aware is a big deal, so as a final plea to everyone, if you remember only one thing from this book: <u>Please pay attention</u>! Pay attention to everything that goes on around you. Be alert and conscious. Focus. Become an arrow of light. Don't piss people off. Be kind all the time. Feed the hungry. Give love freely. Learn to accept things for what they are, and finally, tell someone else. Help them to do the same.

This book has all been about learning to cope with whatever it is you have and set forth from now on to live well.

I bet you never thought this level of sarcasm could be achieved by one man.

If the only thing you can remember to tell your friends about this book is that I dropped a lot of colorful f-bombs; then you failed. I want you to pass. Please, go back and read it again.

So the seed is planted. Vaya con Dios America. The truth is I never left you. All through my wild days - my mad existence. I kept my promise, don't keep your distance.

$20.00
ISBN 978-0-615-31293-4
52000>

9 780615 312934